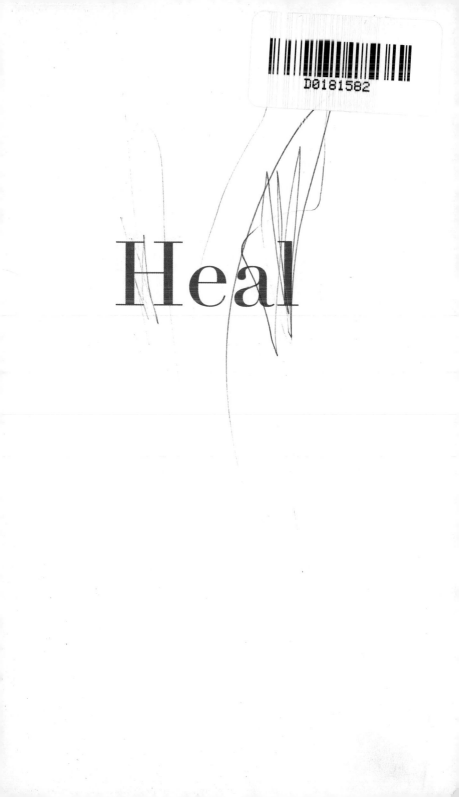

Heal

Heal

THE VITAL ROLE OF DOGS IN THE
SEARCH FOR CANCER CURES

Arlene Weintraub

ECW Press

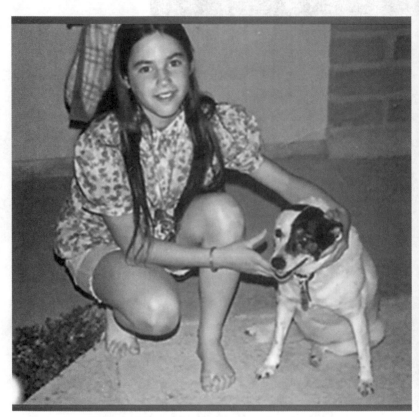

Beth and Spot, the fox terrier mix, circa 1973

For My Family

In Loving Memory of
Beth Ellen Weintraub Schoenfeld,
1962–2010

Contents

Prologue
206 Dogs

In February 2012, I flew to San Francisco, rented a tiny Suzuki four-door sedan, and drove 120 miles southeast in search of inspiration from dogs. I headed for Los Banos, California, home of retired schoolteachers Alan and Kathy Wilber, whose golden retriever, Basil, had been diagnosed with cancer in 2001 at the age of two. In a last-ditch attempt to save their young dog's life, the Wilbers entered Basil into an experimental drug trial.

This trial was part of a growing international effort to recruit dogs with cancer for research designed to yield new and vastly improved treatments — for both man and man's best friend. The scientists who invented that drug were also developing a version of it for people, and using what they learned from the dog trial to improve their efforts.

I had been working as a science reporter when I first learned about this initiative, which is called comparative oncology. Fascinated, I set out to learn as much as I could about the dogs contributing to the search for cancer cures.

My interest was not just professional, nor was it entirely driven by my lifelong love of dogs. Two years before I met Basil's family, I lost my sister, Beth, to gastric cancer. Witnessing her brutal battle against a disease that was ultimately unconquerable left me feeling empty and hopeless. So after she died, I sought comfort in the stories of the dogs whose own cancer battles were inspiring new treatments.

As I dug deeper into the topic, I learned that one of the first big comparative oncology projects was a trial at the University of California at Davis — the trial that offered Basil a second chance at life. That research resulted in Palladia, the first-ever product approved by the Food and Drug Administration (FDA) to treat cancer in dogs,[1] and a similar drug for people called Sutent.

A young veterinary oncologist at UC Davis named Cheryl London conceived of and managed the two clinical trials that the FDA required before it would approve Palladia. The first trial started in 2001 and enrolled fifty-seven dogs whose owners were willing to try the little-understood new drug.[2] That trial was a success and led to a second, more complex research project, involving ten veterinary clinics and 149 dogs.[3]

Among the 206 dogs that nudged Palladia to market were purebreds and mixed breeds, giant dogs and tiny lapdogs. They had one thing in common: their owners were willing to advance the search for a cure in return for the slim chance that they would get to spend more time with their beloved pets.

Ten years later, I wanted to learn more about those 206 dogs and their owners. I knew the dogs were gone, whether they had lost their battle against cancer, or had won it and ended up dying of old age. But I needed to hear their stories and see their photos. I needed to tell their owners that their contribution to cancer research was making a difference for millions of patients and pets around the world. Most of all, I needed to see how the trailblazing research that they had participated in had given rise to other studies that were yielding new therapies for dogs and people with cancer.

I needed 206 reasons to believe there was hope for a cure.

I soon realized, however, that uncovering all 206 stories would not be easy. When I reached London by phone to tell her about my book project, she explained that clinical trial records in veterinary medicine are often thrown out a few years after they're published, which would make it difficult for me to locate the names and contact information for the participants in those trials. Furthermore, many pet owners lose touch with their veterinary oncologists after their dog's treatment has finished — either because the dog survives and returns to a normal, healthy life, or doesn't, and the owner moves on, eager to put the whole cancer nightmare behind them. London simply no longer knew where most of the Palladia trial participants were.

I was undeterred.

My mission turned into a much broader journey, during which I learned about hundreds of research programs aimed at finding new cures for cancers that are the same in dogs and people. As I met the dogs and their owners who were participating in this research, I became more and more curious about exactly how veterinary medicine is helping uncover innovative new pathways in the search for those elusive cures.

So I broadened the boundaries of my research even further. I looked into newly released reports about the dogs' remarkable ability to sniff out cancer and the efforts underway to translate that talent into devices that might be able to detect some cancers in humans before they produce symptoms. Even our feline friends, I learned, are becoming allies in the war on cancer (see Chapter 8).

My story includes information I gathered during visits to eight universities over the course of two years, along with additional details I learned during in-person and telephone interviews with people who participate in comparative oncology research. All of the anecdotes and quotes in this book come from my interviews with veterinarians, oncologists, scientists, drug company executives, and pet owners, unless otherwise noted.

The recollections of the people I talked with are not perfect. But with the help of many experts who are leading the comparative oncology movement, I have done my best to present the events that occurred and the dialogue that was spoken as accurately as possible.

What follows is a story of the quest for healing — of dogs and people suffering from cancer, and of one bereaved sister looking for hope in cancer research.

After Beth began chemotherapy, the basic chores that came with caring for her family's dog, Honey — even the simple act of opening the screen door to let the dog into the backyard — became too much for her. Now, when I let my dog into the backyard I often think about Beth's fight with cancer. With each step toward the back door comes a sad memory, or a twinge of guilt, or a question. How does cancer strike down one member of a family that has virtually no history of the disease? How can a patient who survives a brutal chemo regimen end up dying of the disease anyway? Why can't we spot cancer early, when it's still possible to cure it?

Man's best friend might help us find the answer to those questions, and more.

Chapter 1
"We Believe in Science"

From the moment Alan and Kathy Wilber brought home their new golden retriever, Basil, in October 2000, they knew the dog would fit right in to the menagerie of pets they had been assembling since their three daughters had grown up and moved away. Basil became fast friends with the Wilbers' other two dogs, a petite shepherd mix named Friday and an aging chocolate lab, Chauni, whom Basil doted over like a protective dad.

Basil spent his days romping with Chauni and Friday in the yard of the Wilbers' home in Los Banos, California, and trotting from room to room carrying his favorite toy, a life-sized stuffed duck. Basil stood twenty-nine inches from paws to forehead — six inches taller than the average golden — but he regarded his size as neither an obstacle nor an advantage. Often when Alan sat in his recliner, the dog would join him, hauling his huge body onto the chair, oblivious to the fact that he was far too big to be a lapdog.

Just after New Year's in 2001, the Wilbers noticed a bump on Basil's right hind leg, below his knee. Their vet told them it was probably nothing more than a bruise, but they were worried. Their previous golden retriever, Teddy, had died of cancer, and they couldn't bear the thought of losing another dog to the disease. By that spring the bump had grown, so Kathy brought Basil back to the vet for a biopsy. A few days later, their fears were realized. The two-year-old dog had cancer.

The Wilbers, both schoolteachers, didn't have a lot of extra money to spend on Basil's medical care, but they wanted to give him the best chance of survival. So they set out on a 140-mile drive to the University of California at Davis, home to one of the most advanced veterinary cancer centers in the country. Veterinarians there discovered that the lump was a sarcoma wrapped around the tibia bone. They amputated the leg, and the Wilbers took Basil back to Davis four times over the next six months for infusions of doxorubicin, a standard chemotherapy drug.

Basil quickly adapted to his new life as an amputee. To compensate for the lost leg, he curled his tail around his body as an anchor. He learned to walk effortlessly, centering his left hind leg beneath his body to distribute his seventy-five pounds comfortably across his slender frame. The Wilbers bought a Roadtrek camper, because Basil could jump into it without having to climb any stairs. They carried a small rug with them wherever they went, so the dog could always sit comfortably.

In November 2001, the Wilbers went back to UC Davis for what they believed would be a routine checkup. When they pulled up in front of Davis's veterinary complex, Basil hopped out of the camper and bounded toward the door. His tail wagging, he greeted everyone with an exuberance that belied the seriousness of his disease. He sat calmly through blood tests and CT scans.

After the tests, veterinarian Gillian Dank called the Wilbers into an exam room and delivered the sobering news: Basil's cancer had spread to his lungs. The Wilbers knew that many dog owners in this situation would opt for euthanasia.

Then Dank told them that her colleague, a young veterinary oncologist named Cheryl London, was looking for pet dogs to take part in an innovative study of a powerful experimental drug — a medicine that would come to be called Palladia. Dog owners who enrolled in the study, Dank said, would get the drug at no charge, as well as complimentary veterinary care throughout.

What's more, Basil's cancer — spindle cell sarcoma — was similar to a tumor type found in humans. The research, the Wilbers learned, might benefit people, even if the drug didn't help Basil.

The Wilbers signed Basil up for London's study that day.

———

It was early morning when I set out for Los Banos to visit the Wilbers. As I drove, I thought about the personal tragedy that had sent me on a quest to find hope in the story of Basil. It had been just over two years since I'd lost my sister, Beth, to gastric cancer. She was forty-seven when she died, after a painful and fruitless year of chemotherapy and surgery. Beth left behind a husband, four children, our parents and older brother — and me, the little sister who had idolized her for as long as I could remember.

My shock and sorrow had barely diminished. One day, Beth was an energetic mom, juggling four children's busy schedules while starting her own home-based business, pausing occasionally to sweep the ever-present crumbs and dog hair off the kitchen floor. The next, she was checking in to the hospital with extreme stomach pain, facing a diagnosis that was as baffling as it was tragic. I still could not grasp how my vibrant sister could be struck down so swiftly by a cancer that had never appeared in our family before, and that was exceedingly rare in someone so young.

From the moment Beth was diagnosed, I tried my best to give her hope. It was an unsettling role reversal. After all, she was my big sister, five years my senior. She was the one who had dried my tears at summer camp when I got homesick, entertained my friends at my birthday parties, and offered me advice, whether I asked for it or not. Now I was expected to be the cheerleader. I did not like this new role, but I had to embrace it. So whenever we spoke on the phone or I visited Beth during her treatments, I tried to convince her that she could beat this disease because she was young and strong.

I knew the odds were not in her favor. So did she. And then she was gone.

For me, that last year of Beth's life was a blur of depressing hospital visits, support group meetings, and awkward phone calls from friends who struggled to make sense of this unspeakable tragedy. I diligently showed up to my job as a magazine science reporter but quickly lost all my passion for the latest medical research. Science, after all, had failed my sister. Writing about it had become little more than a sad obligation.

Then two veterinarians from Texas A&M University came to my office to publicize their new, state-of-the-art cancer center, which was designed to find new cures, not just for animals, but for people too. I was surprised to learn that dogs get many of the same cancers we do, including lymphoma, melanoma, breast cancer, bone cancer, and gastric cancer. Texas A&M, they explained, was part of a rapidly expanding network of academic veterinary centers that recruit pets with cancer for "translational" research — studies that have the potential to speed up the search for a cure for humans.

I became enthralled by the idea that research with pet dogs might spare other families from suffering a tragedy like ours. This felt natural. After all, Beth and I were born into a family of dog fanatics. I loved all of them, from Spot, the fox terrier mix who never minded when my sister and I tugged on her tail or tried to dress her in doll clothes, to my treat-loving terrier mix, Molly, whom I nicknamed my midlife crisis dog when I adopted her just after I turned forty. I even bonded with Honey, the lanky, standoffish mutt Beth's family rescued from a shelter when their eldest son turned thirteen.

The veterinarians leading this branch of cancer research work in an emerging field called comparative oncology. The premise of comparative oncology is simple but powerful: Dogs make ideal models for studying human cancer because, like us, they develop cancer naturally. That makes them much more realistic models for human cancers than the rodents that are most commonly used in the discovery and development of new therapies.

Mice and rats rarely develop cancer, so they have to be manipulated in some way to mirror the human cancer experience. Some have tumors implanted under their skin, while others are genetically engineered to be prone to certain types of cancer. Research rodents are often genetic clones whose immune systems are no longer intact. What's more, their diets are tightly controlled, and they live in "clean rooms" that are scrubbed of all the pathogens that we encounter every day.

That may explain why an estimated nine out of ten experimental drugs that cure lab rodents of their cancers fail miserably in human trials.[1] As Richard Klausner, former director of the National Cancer Institute, told the *Los Angeles Times* in 1998, "We have cured mice of cancer for decades — and it simply didn't work in humans."[2]

Our closest animal cousins, non-human primates, are rarely useful in cancer research either. Even though we share more than 90 percent of our genes with them, we are far more susceptible to cancer than they are. Cancers of the breast, prostate, and lung, for example, cause more than 20 percent of human deaths, but occur in less than 2 percent of great apes.[3]

Because of growing international concerns about the ethics of keeping wild animals in captivity purely for medical research, the scientific world has been moving away from primate studies. In June 2013, the National Institutes of Health announced that it would retire most of its laboratory chimpanzees to wildlife sanctuaries.[1] All told, less than 1 percent of all animals used in medical experiments today are primates.[5]

Pet dogs who are stricken with cancer can help fill this void in medical research. About six million dogs are diagnosed with cancer every year in the United States alone.[6] Many of them have forms of the disease that are so similar to ours that even the most eagle-eyed cancer specialists would struggle to tell them apart. As Texas A&M veterinarian Theresa Fossum put it that day she came to my office, "We have access to companion animals with diseases that are genetically identical to their human counterparts."

In comparative oncology, researchers at biotechnology companies team up with veterinary oncologists and with physicians who treat people at cancer centers around the world. They work together to translate discoveries they make in dogs with cancer — perhaps about cancer-causing mutations and how they might be corrected, or new surgical methods for removing tricky tumors — into treatments for people. As they test new drugs or devices or techniques in both dogs and people, they trade insights, with the aim of improving promising treatments and moving them as quickly as possible to the market.

This isn't animal experimentation. Comparative oncology isn't about breeding colonies of cancer-ridden dogs in the lab, and then giving them unproven medications to see how they'll react. The number-one goal of comparative trials, as it is in human clinical trials, is to improve the prognoses for the patients who participate. Fossum explained that the dogs who take part in this research get access to leading-edge treatments and top-notch follow-up care that's often entirely paid for by the companies or research groups funding the trials. Throughout their treatments, the dogs are regarded as valuable members of the scientific team, whose experiences in the trials could pave the way to new cures for cancer.

Scientists working in comparative oncology have been helped by emerging research suggesting that, genetically speaking, our canine companions are more closely related to us than we realize. In 2005, scientists at the Broad Institute, which is co-managed by Harvard University and the Massachusetts Institute of Technology, sequenced the genome of a female boxer named Tasha.[7] They discovered that dogs and people have about 85 percent of the same nucleotides — the molecules that link together to form DNA.

This means the genetic commonalities between dogs and humans are far greater than they are between mice and humans, explained Kerstin Lindblad-Toh, who is the scientific director of vertebrate genome biology at the Broad Institute and one of the co-authors of the paper describing Tasha's genome. Most mammals have about twenty thousand genes, and most of these are similar across species, she said when I reached her by phone to talk about comparative oncology, but it is the nucleotide overlap that's key to determining how closely related one creature is to another. And when it comes to providing a good model for the human experience, dogs rule.

"The regulation of genes — when and how they are turned on and off, what they produce, and so forth — is overall more similar between dogs and humans than it is between mice and humans," Lindblad-Toh said. "That's important for clinical trials. Say you have a drug that's supposed to interact with a certain portion of a protein. It's likely that protein will have the same structure and composition in dogs as it does in humans. Exactly the same." That means the dog is more likely than the mouse to provide an accurate picture of how that drug will work in people.

In addition to sequencing Tasha's genome, the Broad team studied the DNA from ten other dog breeds and compiled a database of millions of genetic components that differ from one breed to another. Since then, scientists there and at other institutions have identified unique genetic markers for dozens of breeds.[8] The result is a treasure trove of genomic data that scientists can use not only to determine what makes some dogs more susceptible to disease than others, but also to better understand the illnesses they share with people and to improve treatments for everyone.

The more I learned about comparative oncology, the more convinced I became of the dog's potential to further the war on cancer. Our companion dogs live in our homes, breathe our air, and eat food grown on our farms and made in our factories, making them susceptible to the same environmental risk factors that contribute to human disease. They bond so closely with us that even though they can't use words to tell us how they're feeling, we know anyway. My dog, Molly, smiles when she's basking in the sun or chomping on her favorite pumpkin chew. And when she needs to expel that gross object she ate off the sidewalk, she freezes, her lips curl, and her eyes take on a glassy gaze. Her expression is exactly what a dog trainer I know calls "barf face."

Our ability to decipher our dogs' emotions and physical well-being is a godsend for veterinary oncologists. They know they can count on pet owners to tell them when the symptoms that alerted them to the cancer go away and their dog starts acting normally again, or when the side effects of a new drug are so harsh he turns his nose up at a favorite treat. Such clues, which are nearly impossible to glean from a mouse in a cage, can help a scientist who has spent years perfecting an experimental treatment to better predict whether it's going to be the next cancer blockbuster or just the latest new idea to bomb in human trials.

Although the Wilbers didn't know it when they enrolled Basil in Cheryl London's trial at UC Davis, their new vet was one of a handful of scientists who were pioneering the field of comparative oncology. After earning her veterinary degree from Tufts University in 1990, London went to Harvard, where in 1999 she earned a Ph.D. in immunology. Then she moved to UC Davis, where she devised trials designed to help both pets and people with cancer.

London was working on Palladia alongside a San Francisco biotechnology start-up called Sugen, which was helping to develop a new class of drugs known as tyrosine kinase inhibitors. These powerful drugs use many different modes of attack against cancer cells. They block a lethal protein produced by a mutation in a gene called c-kit — a gene that had been implicated in some human cancers, including gastrointestinal stromal tumors (GISTs), which originate in the tissue that surrounds the stomach and intestines. That c-kit mutation was also found in some dogs with mast cell tumors, a common form of skin cancer.

In addition to blocking the mutant c-kit protein, Sugen's experimental drugs cut off the blood supply to tumors and slowed down the proliferation of cancer cells by inhibiting two other proteins: vascular endothelial growth factor (VEGF) and platelet-derived growth factor (PDGF).[9]

The effort to develop Palladia began around 2000, when London read a journal article co-written by Gerald McMahon, Sugen's head of drug discovery. London cold-called McMahon and explained to him that the c-kit mutation occurs in some dogs with cancer. She asked him if she could study some of Sugen's tyrosine kinase inhibitors in dogs.

McMahon didn't need much convincing. Two of Sugen's previous tyrosine kinase inhibitors had made tumors shrivel in lab mice, but then failed to produce any meaningful results in human trials. One of the drugs increased the median survival rate of mice with colon cancer by 58 percent — an unqualified success.[10] But when Sugen's scientists tried the same drug in people, it was so poorly absorbed by the body it was bound to have little effect against tumors.[11] McMahon and his colleagues were desperate for a fresh perspective and an opportunity to try the next generation of the drug in something more realistic than a mouse.

McMahon gave London samples of three of the tyrosine kinase inhibitors Sugen was testing, and they planned a study using samples of cancer cells from dogs. London and her colleagues at UC Davis, collaborating with scientists at Sugen, spent the next several weeks drawing the drugs into pipettes, dripping them onto the mutant cells, and watching them under the microscope to see how they reacted.

Each time the result was the same: within forty-eight hours, the cells were either paralyzed or dead.[12]

London selected the most promising of the three drugs and began recruiting dogs for the first trial in March 2001. The drug was developed to target the c-kit mutation common in mast cell tumors, but London and the Sugen team were curious to see if its multi-pronged action might be effective against other types of tumors. Most of all, London wanted to test whether the drug was safe for dogs to take. So she took dogs into the trial who had different cancers: bladder cancer, lymphoma, or sarcomas such as Basil's.

Having lost my sister to gastric cancer, I was particularly fascinated by the Palladia research program, because it had provided key insights for the development of Sutent, a similar tyrosine kinase inhibitor for people. That drug was approved by the U.S. Food and Drug Administration in 2006 to treat some patients with gastrointestinal stromal tumors (GISTs),[13] becoming one of the first genetically targeted treatments approved for that type of gastric cancer.

Gastric cancer is the fifth most prevalent form of the disease, striking about 950,000 patients each year worldwide.[14] It is the third most lethal cancer; only about 30 percent of those diagnosed with the disease live more than five years.[15] That's because gastric cancer is a silent killer — it produces no symptoms until it has spread beyond the stomach, at which point it is nearly impossible to control. By the time Beth was diagnosed, she was in stage four, meaning her cancer had already spread to her lymph nodes.

I knew from writing about the pharmaceutical industry that Sutent was far from perfect. It was so toxic that many patients couldn't take it at all. I also knew that fewer than 5 percent of patients diagnosed with gastric cancer each year had GISTs.[16] My sister was not one of them, as we learned when she was diagnosed a few years after the drug was approved. Her only treatment options were surgery and traditional chemotherapy. Her chances of remission or a cure were slim at best.

Still, I appreciated Sutent's value. The drug worked well in many patients with the c-kit mutation. This was personalized medicine at its best — a drug designed to burrow into some tumors, exploit their genetic weaknesses, and make them melt away. For those few thousand patients diagnosed with GISTs every year, Sutent was a chance for life where there was none before.

And dogs helped make it happen.

———

It was clear I had entered the home of animal lovers the moment I stepped into Alan and Kathy Wilber's kitchen and tripped over two giant dog beds that took up nearly half the floor. Kathy and Alan had retired and now spent much of their spare time volunteering at the local animal shelter, they told me. Basil and his buddies had long since passed, and new pets slept on those dog beds. As I walked in, Hershey, a chocolate Labrador retriever, and Mocha, a yellow Lab, ran up to greet me. Then Hershey dashed off to wrestle with the Wilbers' orange tabby kitten, Stripes, and Mocha grabbed a plush green octopus and took it into the living room to play on his own.

"Our home is just filled with dog beds and toys. It's just who we are," said Kathy, apologizing for the clutter as we navigated around the dogs' beds toward the kitchen table.

Kathy was wearing paw-print earrings that day, and she had covered the table with two giant scrapbooks filled with photos of Basil palling around with the Wilbers' three grown daughters and seven grandchildren. She also brought out the ribbon of appreciation the veterinary school at UC Davis had given to Basil, and a small pile of newspaper and magazine clippings about his role in the Palladia trial.

As Kathy reminisced about Basil, the tears started to flow down her cheeks. Basil, she explained, had been like a child to her and Alan. They were not about to let cancer take him away at such a young age, and they jumped at the chance of trying the new drug.

Basil bonded with his new vet the moment he met her, Alan said. London, petite with cascading brown curls, wasn't that much bigger than her three-legged patient. But she always had a pocketful of treats, and that made her an instant friend of Basil.

"He'd see her and he'd run to her," Alan said. "She had a good rapport with him. She did with all the dogs."

After London enrolled Basil in her trial, she sent the Wilbers home with a bucket of large pills, a sheet of instructions, and strict orders to feed the dog six thousand calories a day — more than double what the average person consumes.

"The dog was going to be eating better than we were," Alan said.

By October 2002, Basil had just three tiny tumors left in his lungs, so UC Davis's team removed two lobes of his lungs.

"Dogs have six lobes, we have four. They have extra lobes here," Alan explained, pointing to his chest, as if he were back at work teaching a class of teenagers.

After the surgery, Basil kept taking Palladia. All this time, the Wilbers were amazed that he never seemed sick. He ate with gusto, and he had plenty of energy for his daily half-mile walks to the park. Alan told me that whenever people stopped them to comment on their three-legged dog, they proudly told them about Basil's participation in cancer research. Alan always took the time to explain that dogs get cancer just like people do, and that veterinarians and doctors were working together to find a cure.

Basil stayed on Palladia until the trial ended in 2004. Every few months, he'd leap out of the back of the Roadtrek camper and run into the vet school for a routine CT scan. One after another, the scans came up clean.

Basil was cured.

Of the fifty-seven dogs who participated in the first Palladia trial, sixteen responded positively to the drug. Six of the dogs, including Basil, saw a "complete response," meaning their cancer disappeared.[17] Basil's lung tumors shrank so dramatically, in fact, that London included his x-rays in the published report on the trial, using an arrow to point to where a once prominent tumor was now a mere blip on the radiograph.

London told me that she had never quite figured out why Basil responded so well to Palladia. He didn't have the c-kit mutation that the drug had proven so adept at targeting. She told the Wilbers that the drug cut off the blood supply to the dog's tumors, and she suspected that's what prompted his long remission. At the time, the concept of inhibiting blood supply to tumors — a process known as anti-angiogenesis — was not fully understood. But it soon became the basis of many successful cancer drugs.

The Wilbers took me on a tour of their modest home, showing me the ramp they built so Basil could easily climb out the doggy door and the articles about him they had framed and hung on the wall. One was a story from the *New York Times*, with a photo of Basil sitting beside Kathy and wearing a scarf that read "CANCER SURVIVOR."

I told the Wilbers that UC Davis was the first veterinary school on my list of schools to visit. I knew I would not meet Cheryl London there, because, in 2005, she left to take a faculty position at the Ohio State University, which had a fledgling comparative oncology program. My itinerary would include London's new home as well as Tufts University, where one vet was collecting tumor samples from dogs with gastric cancer, with the goal of finding new molecular pathways for drugs to fight the disease.

The Wilbers told me their only experience with cancer had come through their dogs. When they enrolled Basil in London's trial, their motive was a simple desire to spend a few more years with him. But the more they learned about London's research, the more reassured they were that they were doing the right thing.

"The advantage of the trial was that it might lead to a drug for humans," Alan said. "That's what kept us going."

Basil spent his healthy years after the study camping with the Wilbers in Oregon and Washington and visiting classrooms to help educate children about careers in veterinary medicine.

After living cancer-free for seven years, Basil developed melanoma in his mouth when he was about nine. His vets determined that the second cancer was completely unrelated to the first. They tried treating it, but the cancer was so advanced no drug would do much to stop it.

Despite everything their dog endured — the loss of a leg and part of his lungs, multiple rounds of an experimental drug, and worst of all, a second cancer — the Wilbers couldn't cite a single regret. When the veterinarians at Davis asked if they could save tissue samples from Basil so researchers in the future might find clues leading to better therapies, the Wilbers readily agreed.

"That's why we put him to sleep at Davis — so they could use him for research," Kathy said. "Hopefully they learned a lot from him."

The Wilbers still felt the Palladia trial had given them an incredible gift.

"The average life for goldens is ten to twelve years. He almost lived out a regular lifespan," Kathy said.

The experimental drug gave Basil seven years of life. As I listened to the Wilbers' stories about their cherished golden, in my head I did the dog math that everyone knows so well: one dog year equals about seven people years. Basil had gained the equivalent of forty-nine people years.

For the first time since Beth died, I wasn't wallowing in my loss. For the first time, I felt a glimmer of hope.

———

On my way to the UC Davis campus, I stopped at the home of Pam Green, whose dog Sweetie participated in the same Palladia trial as Basil. Following Green's directions, I turned down a gravel road and headed through a field of sprawling yellow wildflowers toward what looked like an abandoned shack. I walked around the fence surrounding the structure, searching for the front door. Assuming I was lost, I turned to get back into my car.

Then I saw the sign: "Chez Bouvier."

Green ran a Bouvier rescue organization out of this place, where she lived with three dogs and the thirty-year-old Mercedes she used to shuttle them around. She came out to greet me, dressed in slippers, a purple sweatshirt, and red sweatpants. Green was a middle-aged animal lover who never had children but had been devoted to dozens of Bouviers ever since she fell in love with the breed at age sixteen.

Green escorted me into the dogs' room, a cluttered space outfitted with a crate, three dog beds, and several space heaters humming in unison. Foxie, a large mixed-breed dog, sat in the crate whimpering for attention, while the two Bouviers, Velvet and Grover, ambled restlessly around the perimeter of the tiny room, which Green had set off from the rest of the house with a ripped curtain. I sat on a rocking chair and Velvet leapt to my side. She knocked her head against my arm, until I reached out to stroke her curly gray-and-white coat.

"So, tell me about Sweetie," I said.

Green placed a photo album in my lap and began turning the pages.

"This is Sweetie Pie at the pound. She was scared," said Green, who had a propensity to punctuate her salty speech with long sighs. "There was this look in her eye. I thought, Oh shit, is she going to be a fear biter? A shelter worker helped me put her in the cab of my pickup."

Green told me that Sweetie got over her fears, and the two trained together to compete in sheep herding contests. I flipped through the album, which was filled with photos of Sweetie walking behind a small herd of sheep and navigating a thin wooden beam perched between two posts.

"What was she like, personality-wise?" I asked.

"She was very sweet with people. I gave her the name. It turned out that she was very quarrelsome with other bitches. Not every bitch," Green said with a sigh, "but some."

One day, when Sweetie was eleven years old, Green was rubbing her belly, and her hand passed over a lump. Green took the dog to UC Davis, where she learned that Sweetie had a tumor in one of her mammary glands. Chemotherapy made virtually no dent in the cancer, which spread to Sweetie's lungs, so when Green was offered the chance to join Cheryl London's study, she figured she had nothing to lose.

A couple of weeks after Sweetie started on Palladia, London discovered the dog's tumors had shrunk to half their original size.

"And I'm flying!" Green said, her voice rising in joy. "I had these visions that she's going to be completely cured."

During the trial, Green told me, she volunteered Sweetie for anything that might help London sort out the intricacies of the new drug. She once left the dog at the hospital for twelve hours, so that interns and students could take samples of Sweetie's blood every few hours. That helped London determine exactly how the drug was moving through the dog's body.

"Sweetie was perfectly happy to lie around the room, getting fussed over by residents and students, cajoling them out of part of their lunch," Green said. "The residents probably went hungry the day she was there."

Sweetie died about seven months into the trial — an outcome that I thought might have upset her owner. But Green wasn't bitter at all.

"I figured at the end of it, this drug had probably given Sweetie five or six months she wouldn't have had," Green said.

The math wasn't as impressive as it was for Basil, but I couldn't help doing it anyway as my rented Suzuki rattled down the gravel road away from Green's house — three-and-a-half people years. I understood Green's gratitude. For anyone facing the loss of a loved one to metastatic cancer, even the tiniest drop of time is so much better than nothing at all.

I drove to the Davis campus and headed for the

veterinary school, a gleaming, glass-faced structure that was a splash of modernity against the surrounding brick buildings.

Grateful pet owners built this school. In the early 2000s, UC Davis raised more than $300 million in private donations to update facilities that had become so outdated that the campus risked losing its accreditation and longstanding status as one of the nation's top veterinary schools.[18] Classes there were overcrowded and the buildings so far-flung that students often had to run from academic halls to the veterinary clinic to get to their training sessions on time. The equipment was outdated, and the school's farm animals were kept in a rotting warehouse called the Haring Hall Barn.[19]

During the renovation, Haring Hall was repurposed, and the veterinary department moved to a state-of-the-art facility that included new classrooms, surgery suites to treat horses and livestock, and even a rehab center for injured racehorses. Then the school built a new small-animal clinic — a high-tech complex with a special wing for dogs and cats with cancer.[20] Soon the teaching hospital was treating nearly forty-eight thousand pets and farm animals per year.[21]

To learn more about Palladia I sat down with UC Davis veterinarian and professor Carlos Rodriguez, who had worked with London on the Palladia trials. He explained that, after the first trial, London and her collaborators at Sugen designed a second study concentrating on dogs with mast cell tumors — the skin cancer that's often driven by the c-kit mutation. During the first trial, they had discovered that dogs who had mast cell tumors with the mutation remained stable for a median period of twenty-one weeks, meaning their cancer didn't progress during that time. Dogs that didn't have the mutation had a median time to progression of under four weeks.[22] They set out to determine in the second trial just how effective Palladia might be in dogs with c-kit driven mast cell tumors.

Rodriguez said he took to calling Tuesday "mast cell day," because that was the day reserved for dogs in the trial. Every Tuesday, he would run from one exam room to another, meticulously measuring each tumor to see if it had shrunk, taking photos, drawing blood, checking the dogs' weights, and grilling the owners about any changes in behavior they were seeing.

"I'd tell them, 'If the dog looks at you funny, I want to know about it,'" Rodriguez said.

When I asked Rodriguez if he remembered any remarkable responses to the drug, he told me about a Shar-Pei who entered the trial with a mast cell tumor that was, he said, "hideous."

"What does hideous look like?" I asked.

"Ulcerated, nasty, oozy, disgusting, stinky," he said. "Hideous."

At the Shar Pei's first follow-up visit, Rodriguez barely recognized the dog. The tumor had shrunk, and in a matter of months it had nearly vanished.

"There was nothing," Rodriguez said. "I saw totally normal skin and hair growing. That dog was a complete responder."

After Sutent and Palladia were approved, other companies flocked to UC Davis with ideas for comparative oncology projects. During my visit, Rodriguez told me about eighteen ongoing trials of drugs that might benefit both pets and humans. Two of them were particularly promising.

The first was examining an enzyme-based drug that starved melanomas of a key amino acid. The drug, developed by a San Diego–based biotech start-up called Polaris, had cured three dogs of melanoma, and oncologists at UC Davis's cancer center were preparing to test it on people. (By the end of 2013, the drug had advanced into the late-stage human clinical trials necessary for FDA approval.)

In the second trial, scientists had created an aerosol version of a widely used chemotherapy drug, hoping to find that delivering it straight to the lungs of children with metastatic bone cancer that had spread to their lungs was more effective than injecting the drug into their veins. Rodriguez was so encouraged by what he was seeing in dogs, he predicted oncologists would want to test the breathable drug in children.

"It appears we're doubling the survival of dogs with osteosarcoma with these aerosols," he said. "We're making inroads into survival. It's very exciting."

I wanted to get a different perspective on the potential value of dogs in oncology research — that of the doctors who treat people with cancer. So I drove fifteen miles east to the UC Davis Cancer Center to visit director Ralph W. deVere White, who was also an associate dean of the medical school and a longtime champion of the veterinary school's cancer program.

DeVere White, a jovial Irish urologist, told me he had embarked on a plan to boost the medical school's research capabilities when he arrived in 1984 to chair the urology department. One of his first moves was to persuade the school's provost to convert two nearby abandoned buildings from an old California state fair into labs, where scientists could use high-tech imaging machines and cell-analysis tools.

"Had you done much in comparative oncology before you got here?" I asked.

"Nothing whatsoever," deVere White said.

But he had an ambitious plan: he wanted UC Davis to earn the prestigious "comprehensive cancer center" designation from the National Cancer Institute (NCI) — a label so rarely awarded that, at the time, less than 1 percent of oncology centers in the United States had been granted it. To get the designation, deVere White would have to demonstrate to the NCI that his university not only provided patients with the latest, most advanced treatments, but that physicians and researchers across campus were working together to develop better approaches to detecting, treating, and ultimately curing cancer.

DeVere White said it took him about five minutes to realize what an invaluable resource the university had in the thousands of cats and dogs with spontaneous tumors that arrived at the vet school every year.

When London began planning comparative oncology trials, deVere White encouraged her and introduced her to oncologists at the medical school. The UC Davis Cancer Center was awarded NCI designation in 2002 and the coveted "comprehensive" designation a decade later — a feat deVere White credits largely to London.

"Cheryl put us on the map," he said.

———

During my stay at UC Davis, I squeezed in a visit with the owners of another Palladia dog London had told me about during our initial phone conversation. I drove to Atherton, California, to the home of Mandy Gullick and her husband, Don Morris, who had volunteered Fawn, their sheltie mix, for the first trial of the drug. Fawn was one of only two dogs in the trial with multiple myeloma, a type of blood cancer that had caused lesions to form in her bones and had interfered with her ability to fight off infections.

As Morris shuffled around the living room looking for old albums with photos of Fawn, Gullick began to laugh. Fawn, a cross-eyed pup with a reddish coat, was just the type of dog who made you laugh all the time, she told me.

"She liked to chase and nip people's ankles. She had that herding background," Gullick said. "I think in her previous life she was a motorcycle rider, because she loved motorcycles."

Gullick and Morris brought an insider's perspective to their dog's battle with cancer: they were both scientists who worked in San Francisco's famed biotechnology corridor. They spoke the language of biology as fluently as London and the other vets at UC Davis. To treat Fawn's cancer, they had tried steroids, chemotherapy, even Thalidomide — the anti-nausea drug that was once banned in the United States because it causes birth defects but had found a second life as a treatment for multiple myeloma. Then London told them about the Palladia trial, and they did not hesitate to sign their dog up for it.

"Fawn seemed so young. We had only had her seven years," Gullick said. "We wanted her to have the best treatment. We were willing to do whatever we could to keep her going, as long as she was happy. We believe in science."

We believe in science.

Those words echoed in my ears as Gullick and Morris reminisced about Fawn. *We believe in science.* How wonderful, I thought, that the faith of these two scientists never wavered, even as they watched therapy after therapy fail their treasured companion. How trusting they were to give their dog a drug that was so new the researchers developing it could not fully explain to them how it worked. *We believe in science.*

Gullick and Morris gave Fawn Palladia pills for two years. She suffered few side effects, even though she was also taking two other medications: an osteoporosis drug to prevent her cancer from breaking down her bones, and prednisone, a steroid commonly given along with cancer treatments to prevent inflammation and nausea.

"She got a bit chubby on the prednisone, but that was it," Gullick said.

There was one other notable side effect, this one to Palladia. Fawn's coat changed hue, from red to blonde, as if it had been bleached. This wasn't surprising: in early human trials, tyrosine kinase inhibitors had the same effect on both mice and people.[23] It turns out that the c-kit gene plays an important role in the development of melanocytes, the cells that produce the melanin pigment found in hair, skin, and eyes. When a patient's hair changed color, Sugen's scientists knew their drug was effectively hitting the c-kit target.

Fawn died in 2003. The experimental drug gave the vivacious sheltie two additional years of quality life.

———

I came away from UC Davis with so many new questions; I realized that my short phone call with London hadn't been enough. I needed to sit down with the pioneering veterinarian and learn more about how the Palladia trials had helped guide the effort to develop a new cancer drug for people. I didn't expect her to tell me that dogs were pointing the way to a miraculous cure for cancer. The year I'd spent watching my sister waste away had taught me not to be overly optimistic.

Still, I believed London's answers to my questions might provide the hope I was looking for in cancer research. I wanted to ask her: How did the different experiences of Basil, Sweetie, and Fawn add to the world's understanding of tyrosine kinase inhibition, the c-kit mutation, and the value of choking off the blood supply to tumors? How did she share the lessons she learned from the Palladia dogs with the scientists working on the human version of the drug? And what other trials in comparative oncology had Palladia inspired her to launch?

I wanted to believe in science, too. For my sister and the countless other people whose lives were stolen way too early by this relentless disease, I needed to hear London tell me that the science of dogs — and all that we share with them — might bring the dream of a cure for cancer a little closer to reality.

Before I left UC Davis, I walked around the gardens surrounding the veterinary cancer center and came across a dog park fenced off by black iron railings. In front of the gate sat a colorful stone, affixed with a plaque, one of many memorials in the park to long-lost pets. I stepped inside the park gingerly, overcome by the feeling that I was somehow disturbing the spirits of all the pets who had been treated here.

Then I saw a small red stone, inscribed in simple, black lettering, "In Loving Memory of Basil Wilber." The memorial concluded with the nickname chosen by London to immortalize the resilient golden retriever, whose stunning response to Palladia helped set the drug on the path to approval.

"MIRACLE DOG."

Chapter 2

Dogs Point the Way
to Personalized Medicine

Katie was a golden retriever with a troubled past who had finally found a good home in El Dorado County, California, when, in 2002, a lump appeared in one of her mammary glands. Katie's owner, Carla McCreary, drove the dog to UC Davis's veterinary school, where she learned the lump was a rare and highly aggressive sarcoma. Surgery and chemo helped shrink the tumor, but then London discovered the cancer had spread to Katie's lungs. She offered McCreary the opportunity to participate in the Palladia trial, explaining that even if the drug didn't help Katie — and it was unlikely it would — the knowledge gained from her experience might someday make a difference for people.

The Palladia worked, and Katie became the trial's second miracle dog. Her lung tumors shrank, and after nine months they were so small that vets at the university were able to remove the two affected lobes. Katie was cured.

I spoke to McCreary by phone after I returned from UC Davis, and she confessed that helping people had not been her priority when she said yes to the Palladia trial.

"It would be nice to say it was purely humanitarian, but all I wanted was to save Katie," she said.

Katie was a habitual runaway who had been found on the streets nurturing a litter of puppies, said McCreary, who worked as the manager of a minimart near her home. A local rescue group adopted out the puppies but struggled to place Katie because of her tendency to flee from people. McCreary and her husband, Mike, eagerly took on the challenge, and worked patiently to earn Katie's trust.

"Katie was truly a con artist," McCreary said. "One of the hardest things about her early life is that she wouldn't bond with people. She loved other animals, but people pretty much disappointed her."

As the dog started to come out of her shell, Carla and Mike enrolled her in obedience training, and then in a program that trained dogs to be pet therapists at hospitals, nursing homes, and shelters. After she won her cancer battle, Katie returned to her work as a therapy dog.

Katie was a star at Children's Receiving Home of Sacramento, a shelter for families that were victims of abuse. On her first visit to the home, McCreary recalled, Katie trotted across a room full of children and climbed onto the lap of a boy who had not smiled or spoken since he had arrived there a week earlier. Suddenly the boy started laughing and regaling the other children with stories of his favorite dogs. Every time Carla took Katie back to the home, the dog seemed to sense where she could bring the most cheer, whether it was playing tug-of-war with a group of boys, or letting a little girl braid her long fur.

"That was her gift — to nurture," McCreary said.

Katie had been cancer-free for nearly two years when Mike was diagnosed with stage four pancreatic cancer and given just months to live. Katie refused to leave his bedside, keeping vigil there, providing him comfort with her presence, until the day he died. Then, just a couple of weeks later, McCreary woke up and was surprised to find that Katie wasn't in the bed beside her. She ran downstairs and discovered that the dog had passed away in her sleep.

McCreary brought Katie's body back to UC Davis, where London determined that she had died of a twisted intestine that was unrelated to her cancer battle. The dog had outrun her risky life on the streets and the disease that should have killed her, passing peacefully at age nine.

Several years later, McCreary was talking with a friend who was fighting cancer. He described a new drug he was taking — a smart drug, he called it — that targeted certain types of tumors.

"The more we talked, the more I thought that had to be a derivative of the drug Katie was on," McCreary said.

Indeed, McCreary's friend was taking Sutent, the tyrosine kinase inhibitor that Sugen developed for people with the help of the insights gained from the Palladia trial. He lived three years beyond his diagnosis, McCreary said.

Katie the nurturer had, in her own small way, helped a family friend — and demonstrated to McCreary the humanitarian value of the Palladia trial that McCreary had initially overlooked.

"For years there was just no hope. But now there's this drug on the market that gave my friend remarkable success and a really good quality of life," McCreary said. "Katie gave back way more than she was given."

———

By the time I flew from New York to Columbus to meet Cheryl London in person at Ohio State University, I'd realized the veterinarian had taken on an almost mythical stature in my mind. I was filled with nervous anticipation, knowing I would soon be face-to-face with the woman who had persuaded the oncology-research community that man's best friend could help cure one of man's greatest scourges.

As I drove from my hotel to the campus, I passed the Horseshoe, Ohio State's giant stadium — a reminder that this school is much better known for its Buckeyes football team than it is for oncology research. Then I checked in for my visit to the veterinary school and was handed a packet filled with medical literature. I reached in and pulled out a red magnet advertising the school's twenty-four-hour veterinary services. It was only a token, but it showed that the scientists and clinicians in this corner of campus had their own version of the school's renowned "Buckeye pride."

Ohio State's veterinary school has a strong legacy of research: Its achievements include developing and patenting the first feline leukemia vaccine in the early 1980s.[1] I was introduced to the school by William Kisseberth, a soft-spoken veterinarian who led the university's comparative oncology effort. He told me that when he came to Ohio State in 2001, there was only one veterinary oncologist on the faculty. Over the next ten years, the school worked hard to build up its oncology practice — an effort that included luring London away from UC Davis in 2005. By the time I visited, the veterinary school was treating thirty-five thousand animals per year, including dogs with cancer from all over the state, and it was running as many as ten oncology studies at a time.

My tour included a visit to the school's canine blood bank, where blood was collected from healthy dogs and sent to veterinary surgical centers all over the country. I was also shown rehabilitation suites filled with exercise gear, including treadmills and giant pools, which creatures from toy poodles to horses could use to regain their strength after surgery. In the large-animal clinic, we passed a long row of stalls filled with horses, and the cow mover — a chute-like vehicle that the vets and their students used to transport their lumbering patients between the treatment rooms and the waiting areas. Elsie, a black and white cat who patrolled the barns each night to keep mice at bay, was playing with the receptionists in the front entry hall.

Inside the companion-animal cancer center's chemo-therapy room, a golden retriever, a Labrador retriever, and a Chihuahua waited patiently in stacked cages for their treatments to begin. A fourth dog, a big black mutt, was lounging on a red bed before his turn in the chemo suite. The golden's fur had been thinned by the chemotherapy he was getting to treat his lymphoma, but he wagged his tail when a vet technician reached for one of two treat jars.

I figured if there was any place a dog would dread, it would be here, but these dogs were cheerful and engaged, playing with the technicians and begging for the next treat. One vet tech explained to me that her job was not just to dole out medicine, but also to make sure every patient there continued to enjoy a dog's life, complete with belly rubs, walks, and treats galore.

This was an important element of the ethical framework within which comparative oncologists worked — a code of conduct that was starting to come alive for me as I traveled from one veterinary school to another. For these clinicians, the need to keep their canine patients happy, and to ensure that the experimental cancer treatments were not causing undue pain and suffering, trumped the search for a cure.

In a small room off to the side, London and two staff members prepared to bring one of the dogs in for chemotherapy. I waited for her to take a break, and we sat down in one of the clinic's exam rooms to talk. I started by asking her the question that had been on my mind since I first heard about her work.

"Why cancer?" I asked.

I had often wondered how health care providers involved in the search for a cancer cure handle the sheer desperateness of trying to conquer the disease — the knowledge that no matter how hard they tried, the tumors would likely outsmart them in the end. This conundrum seemed to be especially challenging in veterinary medicine. After all, London's four-legged patients couldn't use words to tell her how they were feeling. They could not voice their opinions about the treatments she was choosing for them. And more often than not, their owners chose euthanasia over the uncertainty and expense of cancer treatments.

Why, I wondered, would anyone choose a career so filled with despair and death?

London told me she was born and raised in Boston and had loved animals for as long as she could remember. But as a child, her allergies were so severe the only pets her mom would let her have were gerbils. She eventually outgrew the allergies and set out to fulfill her dream of becoming a veterinarian. She was the type of kid who liked to search for order in disorder, often taking apart radios just for the challenge of figuring out how to put them back together. As an undergraduate, she chose to study developmental biology and was almost immediately drawn to the puzzle of cancer.

"I saw cancer as development gone awry — the opposite of order," she said.

I asked London to tell me more about how Palladia advanced from idea to finished drug. From the beginning, she said, she coordinated closely with Sugen, frequently offering up insights she'd gleaned from the dog trial to the scientists working on the human form of the drug.

For example, London noticed that some dogs on Palladia who used to run happily into the clinic were now stopping short on the lawn in front, walking gingerly and refusing to step on the sidewalk that led to the front door. She deduced that the dogs were probably suffering muscle aches that made it painful for them to walk on hard surfaces. When she mentioned this to Sugen's scientists, they told her that some people in early trials of Sutent were complaining of similar problems.

So London dropped the dosage in the Palladia trial,

instructing the dog owners to give the pills every other day instead of every day. In no time, the dogs stopped shying away from sidewalks and roads. They walked normally again — a sure sign that the pain had diminished. Surprisingly, the drug seemed to maintain its tumor-killing capability at the smaller dose.

Dirk Mendel, who led the development of Sutent, told me he found the exchanges with London invaluable.

"It gave us a lot of confidence," said Mendel, who had moved on to a job with the pharmaceutical company MedImmune when I talked to him about Sutent. "We saw an opportunity to show very broad, very good anti-tumor activity with this drug."

For human patients with GIST stomach cancer, the discovery of the c-kit mutation targeted by drugs like Palladia and Sutent was revolutionary. A group of Japanese scientists first described the mutation in 1998.[2] A few years later, a tyrosine kinase inhibitor that could block c-kit, a Novartis drug called Gleevec, came onto the market in the United States, approved first to treat a form of leukemia and later to treat GIST.

Oncologists at the Dana-Farber Cancer Institute at Harvard University in Cambridge, Massachusetts, helped conduct the clinical trials for both Gleevec and Sutent, and it didn't take long for them to understand the value of being able to combat genetic mutations with drugs.

"This was the first personalized, targeted therapy for the treatment of solid tumors," said Suzanne George, clinical director of Dana-Farber's Center for Sarcoma and Bone Oncology, when I reached her by phone. "Now we had a solid tumor with a specific driving mutation, and if we blocked it with a drug, we could shut down the disease."

But there was a problem: GIST, which is a type of sarcoma, kept escaping Gleevec's grip, often by developing secondary mutations that the drug was powerless to block. Patients in the trials invariably became resistant to Gleevec, and their tumors came roaring back. Sutent was able to inhibit some of those secondary mutations, and it also seemed to be effective in the small proportion of GIST patients who didn't have the c-kit mutation. Adding Sutent to the toolbox made the potential for long-term survival with GIST more than a distant dream.

"Before these drugs, the average survival for metastatic GIST was around a year," George said. "Now it's at least five years. Resistance is still a challenge, but this was a very dramatic change in the paradigm of the disease."

For London, who was driven mostly by the desire to help animals with cancer, guiding Palladia to market was far from easy. The drug giant Pharmacia had acquired Sugen in 1999 and was integrating the start-up into the larger corporation just as the first Palladia trial was getting underway. Suddenly London was thrown into the world of Big Pharma, where the desire to make a profit and keep shareholders happy competes with the drive to develop innovative new therapies.

Sutent continued to advance through the development process at Pharmacia, but Palladia stalled. Although Pharmacia was a leader in the animal health industry, it didn't have any experience in developing drugs to treat pets with cancer, and its marketing executives weren't convinced there would be enough deep-pocketed pet owners willing to buy Palladia for their ailing dogs.

"Everyone was trying to decide whether or not this was going to be a drug that was going to make money," London said. "It was a challenging time."

———

We were halfway through our chat when London was called away to consult with the owners of one of the dogs she was treating. While I waited for her to return, assistant professor Sandra Barnard came into the room to tell me about her work. Barnard was a native of Australia, who earned her veterinary degree at the University of Sydney before coming to the United States for a residency at Cornell. She was planning to return to Australia in 2013, after a brief stint at Ohio State to learn how to conduct cancer trials in pets.

When I asked Barnard what her cancer specialty was, her response surprised me.

"Communications," she said.

Barnard had become adept at teaching veterinary students how to talk to pet owners about cancer treatments and clinical trials.

"I feel communication is essential," she said, "especially in oncology, when we're dealing with end-of-life — a terminal disease."

With the blessing of pet owners, the veterinary clinic videotaped discussions between students and incoming clients. Then, every Friday, Barnard watched the tapes with the students, pointing out where they might have been more empathetic, or perhaps could have better explained what would happen if the owners enrolled their dog in a particular trial.

Barnard asked me what inspired me to write a book about dogs with cancer. I told her about my sister, our mutual love of dogs, and my search for consolation in comparative oncology.

"This is a good place to find hope, right?" I said.

Barnard nodded, then asked, "How did you feel you were treated during your sister's experience?"

My sister was diagnosed and treated in Israel, where she had lived for more than twenty years. Israel is home to some of the world's top gastric cancer specialists, and we knew Beth was getting the best care available. But experiencing her cancer from afar — dealing with doctors who conduct their business in a language I don't speak, never quite grasping the particulars of her disease or prognosis — was alienating, frustrating, and often terrifying.

I explained to Barnard that Beth's doctors hadn't given us much reason for optimism.

"There was nothing they could do except torture her with chemotherapy and surgery," I said.

After Beth completed her chemo treatments, she underwent a surgery so radical only a few physicians in the world would even attempt it. Her surgeon removed most of her stomach, spleen, part of her colon, and several cancerous lymph nodes found near the tumor site in a last-ditch effort to stop the disease from taking over her body.

A few days later, Beth's surgeons sent her home. But she could not eat. Not the boiled eggs her doctor begged her to try. Not the milky drinks that were supposed to provide much-needed nutrition. Beth would not touch them. She described a confounding combination of hunger and fullness, of feeling simultaneously ravenous and so nauseated she couldn't bear to let anything pass her lips. A few days after arriving home, Beth was back in the hospital hooked up to an IV drip that provided the nutrition she needed.

I had visited Israel earlier to help Beth and her family during her chemo treatments, but I knew I had to go back. I took a short leave from my job, flew to Tel Aviv, and went straight to Beth's hospital, a sprawling medical campus with a grand piano in the lobby. Our mother had e-mailed me precise directions to Beth's room, but when I got there, I thought I must have made a wrong turn at the piano or ventured into the wrong set of elevators. On the bed inside the room there was an old woman with short, gray hair, lying on her side, her back to the door. I turned away and began walking around the circular hallway, peeking into each room, looking for Beth.

Then I realized that old woman who had turned her back on the world was my sister. I went into her room and sat on her bed. She reached for my hand.

"Thank you for coming," Beth said, in a voice I could barely hear.

One afternoon, as I sat with her, begging her to eat, a surgeon marched into her room with a handful of residents, and gestured to me to leave. I sat outside, watching the doctors stand at the foot of Beth's bed and jabber to each other in Hebrew. A few minutes later the doctors left, and I went back into the room.

"He called me an experiment," Beth said, turning toward the wall and curling herself into a dejected ball.

I searched my brain for words to comfort her — words to soften the sting of *that* word, the cold and sterile "experiment." Nothing came to me.

I knew what that surgeon was saying: Six rounds of chemotherapy had shrunk the stomach tumor, but none of Beth's doctors could promise her that the surgery had eradicated the rest, nor could they predict whether the procedure itself might make her sicker than the cancer and chemotherapy already had. Still, I wanted to run out of the room, find that surgeon, and scream at him.

How could he call a living person an experiment? Did he kick me out of the room because he knew that what he was saying was wrong, and he didn't want her family to know how unsure he was that this surgery would work? Didn't anyone ever teach him that patients are fragile, and that they need their physicians to speak to them with kindness and understanding?

I was comforted to learn from Barnard that, at least in the world of veterinary medicine, clinicians understand the importance of empathy.

Much of Barnard's work — and the message she planned to take back with her to Australia — centered on teaching young veterinarians that they shouldn't keep pets on experimental treatments unless they were sure the medicines were making a difference and the animals were enjoying a good quality of life while being treated. For most veterinarians, this was common sense, but helping pet owners through the process of letting go when a dog was not benefiting from the trial was far from easy.

Barnard told me about one dog who had to be taken off an experimental drug because it wasn't working, and it was making the dog sicker than before. His owner didn't agree with the decision.

"She was so angry that we stopped the drug," Barnard said. "I think part of it was she felt we were giving up. But really, it's not fair for a dog to die feeling crappy."

This desire to prioritize patient comfort over science seemed to distinguish comparative oncology from other types of animal research, both practically and ethically. As I got further into my research, I wanted to know more about what ethicists thought of the growing field of comparative oncology. Did they examine this research with the same scrutiny given to scientists who perform experiments on laboratory animals such as mice, rats, and the colonies of beagles and other dogs that are used solely to test medical products? In search of answers, I called Andrew Rowan, chief executive officer of Humane Society International, chief scientific officer of the organization's American branch, and an authority on the ethics of animal research.

Rowan told me that the best way to approach the subject is not to lump comparative oncology in with traditional animal research, which is never aimed at helping the animals. Rather, comparative studies should be thought of more like human clinical trials that involve patients who are not competent enough to make their own decisions about participating in the research, either because they're children or because they are adults who are mentally impaired.

Pets are equally treasured, Rowan said, and they rely

on their owners to determine what's best for them. "They have a family who loves them, but they're not capable of giving what is known as informed consent."

That means it's up to the pet owner — just as it would be up to a parent or guardian — to decide whether participation in a clinical trial is a good idea. And it's the responsibility of the veterinarians to tell pet owners when they feel that the trial is no longer in the best interests of the animal.

Once the veterinarian quells any concerns about suffering, Rowan said, the only ethical question worth fretting over is the same quandary that plagues every human clinical trial ever conducted: What if the research fails to produce any meaningful advancements in the search for a cure? Is participating in the trial still worth it?

"Part of the problem in the whole research endeavor is that it's difficult to identify what the benefits will be," Rowan said.

He compared scientific research to building a house, with every clinical trial as a brick. No one can predict whether any single brick will ultimately be part of a beautiful home, or whether someone might come along, decide it's all wrong, topple the bricks with a bulldozer, and start over again.

"Most of science is bricklaying," Rowan said. "But we don't know which brick is going to create the revolution."

He told me that the Humane Society supported comparative oncology and all other clinical research designed to help animals, and that it has made great strides in its efforts to reduce the reliance on lab animals in human drug development. For example, it launched a protest against the drug company Allergan, which had for years used mice to test each batch of its famed anti-wrinkle drug, Botox, for proper potency. The testing caused many of the mice to suffocate to death. In 2011, after nearly a decade of pressure from the Humane Society, Allergan introduced an animal-free, fully automated Botox test.[3]

Technology has been replacing lab animals so rapidly that Rowan offered the bold prediction that the use of lab animals for safety testing in drug development will end completely by 2025.

———

After Pharmacia swallowed up Sugen, casting a cloud over the prospects for Palladia, London vowed to do whatever she could to make sure the project stayed alive. In winter 2002, when London's first Palladia trial was in full swing, Pharmacia invited her and several other veterinarians to the company's headquarters in Kalamazoo, Michigan, for a meeting to discuss whether there would be enough demand for Palladia to justify further investment in its development. The company's cavernous conference room was filled with Pharmacia's marketing staff, along with a handful of people from its animal health division.

Among those who attended the meeting was a towering, dour-faced Dutchman named Folkert Kamphuis. As Pharmacia's head of global marketing, he was the executive who would ultimately determine whether the company should pursue FDA approval for Palladia, and he went into the meeting feeling skeptical.

After London gave an overview of the science behind Palladia, Kathy Mitchener, a veterinarian in Memphis, took the floor. Mitchener was well known on the lecture circuit for her engaging presentations on how general veterinary practitioners could incorporate oncology treatments into their practices. She told stories about the dogs who had visited her oncology clinic and the owners who paid thousands of dollars to treat their pets.

After Mitchener finished her talk, Kamphuis strode up to her, and said, "I want to visit your practice."

A week later, the Pharmacia executive boarded a plane to Memphis.

When I called Kamphuis to get more of the Palladia story, he told me that after he arrived at Mitchener's Angel Care Cancer Clinic, Mitchener sat him down in an exam room filled with soft chairs and a comfortable couch. She had spent the previous week calling her clients and asking them to come to the clinic to meet with Kamphuis and tell him their stories. A few had already lost their pets to the disease, but most were still waging the battle. Many of their dogs suffered from mast cell tumors — the tumor type that would ultimately become the main target of London's Palladia research.

One of Mitchener's clients was a lighting designer for rock concerts, Kamphuis recalled, who lived with his dog in an old, painted Volkswagen van. He told Kamphuis that he had come back to Memphis from California because he couldn't find a veterinary oncology clinic as good as Mitchener's there. One woman, whose dog had died a month earlier, told Kamphuis she took out a second mortgage on her home to pay for her pet's cancer treatments. Then there was the man who went for a run every day with his dog, until the dog started limping. It turned out to be bone cancer, which was cured with amputation. The man and his dog were running together again.

Mitchener had booked twenty clients to meet with Kamphuis that day, but after speaking with just five of them, the Pharmacia executive burst out of the room with tears streaming down his face.

"I can't take this anymore," he told Mitchener.

She cajoled him back into the room, explaining patiently that he needed to hear all the stories to understand why the veterinary world needed drugs like Palladia. Kamphuis met all twenty clients that day and a few more the next.

"It was fascinating to see the passion of these people and the extent of the sacrifices they would make to pay for treatments for their pets," said Kamphuis, who by the time I spoke to him had moved to a new job at Novartis. "It was an emotional day."

As Kamphuis prepared to return to Kalamazoo, he looked Mitchener in the eyes and made her a promise.

"You will have your drug."

A few months later, pharmaceutical giant Pfizer bought Pharmacia and continued to invest in developing both Palladia and Sutent. Based on the rapidly expanding understanding of c-kit and the experiences in the first trial, Pfizer decided to develop the drug for the treatment of dogs with mast cell tumors that carried the mutation. So it launched a second, pivotal trial of Palladia on dogs with mast cell tumors, which was managed by London, Mitchener, and veterinarians at eight other clinics.[4]

I spoke to former Pfizer scientists Steven Kamerling and Gina Michels, who took many of the insights they gained from London's initial study to determine, for example, the best dose of Palladia to test in a larger mast-cell trial. By the time I spoke with them, they were working for Zoetis, an animal health company that was spun off from Pfizer in 2013, but their memories of London's dedication — and that of the pet owners who volunteered for the trials — were still fresh.

"Each time [the dog owners] gave the drug they were required to write that down. And if the dog were to spit a pill out, they had to report that, too," Michels said. "They had to come back for regularly scheduled visits. They were also responsible for reporting any adverse side effects to their veterinarians. It took a big commitment from the pet owners."

After six years of research and multiple meetings with the FDA, Palladia was finally approved for dogs in June 2009. Pfizer took all the information it had gathered from patients, their owners and veterinarians, and used it to develop the label and prescribing information that came with the drug, Michels said.

Despite all the excitement of the FDA approval, veterinarians would soon see that Palladia was far from a cure-all for mast cell tumors. During the second trial, 43 percent of the dogs receiving Palladia responded positively, but the drug delayed tumor progression in those dogs by an average of just eighteen weeks. The researchers did show that the presence of the c-kit mutation mattered: 60 percent of the dogs in the first phase of the trial who received the drug and had the mutation experienced some positive response, versus just 20 percent of dogs who didn't have the mutation.[5] Still, removing mast cell tumors surgically was the most widely accepted treatment method, and it wasn't clear Palladia offered enough advantages to compete with that.

Because of those caveats — and the fact that Palladia was the first cancer drug ever approved by the FDA to treat pets — veterinary oncologists would need some convincing. So Pfizer held a series of educational webinars for veterinary professionals, giving free samples of the drug to anyone who completed the program.

"Pfizer had a very smart development plan," London said. "They recognized they weren't going to be successful unless they had the buy-in from the oncology folks."

Although London was sometimes frustrated by the constant changes that came first with the Pharmacia takeover and then the Pfizer buyout, she had come to respect Pfizer's expertise and the great care they took bringing Palladia to market.

After Palladia was approved, other companies began contacting London to learn more about how companion dogs might help them in developing new drugs. At the time of my visit to Ohio State University, she was working with a Boston-based biotech company called Karyopharm Therapeutics, which had invented a set of compounds that inhibit a protein called CRM1. In healthy people, proteins in the center of each cell work constantly to prevent those cells from becoming cancerous. But sometimes CRM1 takes over and pushes those tumor-suppressing proteins out of the cells, allowing tumors to form.

Karyopharm asked the vets at Ohio State to test an early iteration of their lead drug in dogs with lymphoma. One of the first dog owners to volunteer was London herself. Her nine-year-old adopted foxhound, George, was suffering from lymphoma, and London hoped the new drug would help keep the cancer at bay.

"George was the world's best dog who was also the world's worst dog," said London, laughing. "He would destroy things in my house. He ate my bedroom door. He ate the banister. There were teeth marks on every piece of furniture."

George was doing well on the drug when suddenly the dog who used to devour everything in sight stopped eating. Even when London gave him drugs to stimulate his appetite, he would not eat.

"I was incredibly frustrated," she said. "I was force-feeding him. It took a while for his appetite to come back."

The scientists at Karyopharm had noticed that the drug ruined the appetites of the mice in their early lab trials, too, but they didn't know why. When London reported the side effect in George and the other dogs in the trial, they realized they had a problem.

London stopped the trial, then restarted it, this time giving the dogs a much lower dose. She increased the dose gradually, until she found the level that worked but didn't affect the dogs' appetites so drastically. In an initial small trial, nine out of fourteen dogs with non-Hodgkin's lymphoma responded well to the drug, charting a median time to progression — the period in which their cancer did not worsen — of sixty-six days.[6]

Inspired by Palladia, Karyopharm worked to develop two versions of its drug in parallel — one for dogs, which it called Verdinexor, and a slightly different formulation for people, named Selinexor. The company worked with London to come up with a steroid-based regimen for offsetting the appetite issues in dogs. By mid-2014, Karyopharm had advanced toward late-stage trials of Verdinexor to treat lymphoma in dogs. The FDA approved the drug for "minor use," meaning Karyopharm could provide it to veterinarians on a select basis to use against canine cancer while completing the pivotal trials required for full approval.[7]

London's work helped Karyopharm design its human trials of Selinexor, one of which took place at Ohio State's James Cancer Hospital and Solove Research Institute.[8]

George didn't survive — he died of heart failure tied to a chemotherapy drug he had taken prior to the Karyopharm trial — but London was eternally grateful to the mischievous dog for helping her prove the value of comparative oncology.

"There's an overwhelming degree of complexity to cancer that is only beginning to be appreciated," London said. "The challenge on the human side is that the mouse models are set up to succeed. You have a cell line or a tumor that's got a mutation, and you inhibit that mutation, and the tumors shrink. But in the reality of human disease, there's far more heterogeneity."

Karyopharm CEO Michael Kauffman told me much of the value of the drug trials with dogs comes from the insights offered by owners. It is their ability to understand how the dogs are feeling that makes all the difference.

"Knowing what this drug does in dogs is immeasurably beneficial," Kauffman said. "We have no idea with rats and mice, frankly. They're caged. It's a very artificial situation. Dogs are in domestic situations. Their owners are extremely attentive."

Some of London's discoveries in dogs came purely through happenstance. When I met her, she was also working with a Boston company called Synta to develop drugs that inhibit heat shock proteins, which, as their name suggests, are proteins produced by both humans and dogs in response to sudden temperature spikes. These proteins seem to play a role in the proliferation of cancerous cells. Synta originally designed its drug to be infused into a vein, but when London tested the technique in dogs, it didn't work.

One day during the trial, a high-strung Belgian Tervuren, who was being treated for melanoma, yanked the catheter out of his vein, and the experimental drug ended up soaking into his skin. London was concerned, because she didn't know how the drug would act outside of the vein.

She soon had an answer. The rowdy dog was the only one in the trial whose cancer shrank. London deduced that delivering the drug under the skin rather than intravenously completely changed how it worked, though she didn't know how. So she designed a new trial, during which her team infused Synta's drug under the skin of dogs with cancer. They all got better.

London went to the company and urged them to reconsider the method they were using to administer the drug. Synta took her advice and went back to the drawing board to devise an alternative dosing strategy, which it later explored in human trials, London said. And it was all because of the Belgian Tervuren who couldn't sit still.

"This," said London, "is science as serendipity."

In the time since Sutent went on the market, it had become a cancer blockbuster, used around the world to treat GIST tumors and some patients with kidney and pancreatic cancer. It was bringing in more than $1 billion in sales for Pfizer per year. And veterinarians were not only using Palladia to treat mast cell tumors, they sometimes tried it on other cancers, in the hope that the drug's ability to deprive tumors of their blood supply would prove effective here as well.

London wanted to prove Palladia would work on more than just mast cell tumors, so she launched trials of the drug with dogs who had several other tumor types. In some trials, she combined the drug with radiation to see if that would make it more potent. In 2012, she published her findings, which provided evidence that Palladia might be effective in treating osteosarcoma, head and neck cancer, and tumors of the anal sacs, thyroid, and nasal cavity.[9] By 2014, she was managing simultaneous studies of Palladia in other tumor types and examining the drug to see if it could inhibit a tumor-promoting protein called janus kinase (JAK).

I told London that meeting the owners of the Palladia dogs had been comforting for me in the wake of my sister's loss, and asked her if losing so many of the dogs she had taken care of ever made her question her career choice.

London's answer harkened back to Basil, Katie, and the other dogs she had cured with drugs that were at the leading edge of scientific discovery. The disappointments and losses, she said, never outweighed the satisfaction of contributing knowledge to a field of science so desperately in need of new ideas.

"The joy for me is in seeing a drug do something phenomenal," she said. "The science — it's just amazing."

Chapter 3
"Do Dogs Get Melanoma?"

In 1999, veterinarian Philip Bergman had just finished his Ph.D. when he was offered the opportunity to help bring Palladia to market. Bergman had recently taken a position as chief of the Donaldson-Atwood Cancer Center at the Animal Medical Center in New York when he got a call from a trial coordinator at Pharmacia. The coordinator asked if Bergman would help recruit dogs with mast cell tumors for the pivotal trial of Palladia that would be required for FDA approval.

Bergman didn't hesitate to sign up for the job. While he was completing his Ph.D. fellowship at MD Anderson Cancer Center in Houston (where he studied human cancer biology so he could better understand the disease that he planned to specialize in as a veterinarian), oncologists were buzzing about the emerging class of tyrosine kinase inhibitors and their potential to revolutionize cancer treatment. Besides, Bergman was eager to help develop a cancer drug designed for dogs, so veterinarians like him would have an alternative to the chemo drugs that had been developed for people.

Just as the pivotal Palladia trial was getting underway that fall, Bergman got a second, quite serendipitous chance to help develop a completely new class of cancer drugs. He was attending a dinner for cancer researchers at the Princeton Club in New York, when a man at his table turned to him and asked, "Do dogs get melanoma?"

That man was Jedd D. Wolchok, an oncologist who specialized in treating melanoma at Memorial Sloan Kettering Cancer Center in New York. Wolchok was developing a new approach to treating melanoma — a vaccine, not to prevent cancer, but to mobilize patients' own immune systems to fight the melanoma already in their bodies. He and his colleagues had collected some promising results from lab rodents, but Wolchok wanted to see if the approach would work in a more realistic model of the disease.

There is no better model for human melanoma than the dog. Melanoma, the most dangerous form of skin cancer, is so similar in dogs and people that if you were to put a melanoma sample from each species under a microscope and challenge a room full of cancer experts to identify which was which, most of them would have to guess. Bergman tried that once, at a conference for human and veterinary pathologists organized by the National Institutes of Health in Bethesda, Maryland.

Bergman explained when I met him that because of subtle but visible distinctions between human and canine skin, "If there had been a piece of [healthy] skin attached to the tumor sample, they would have been able to tell the difference. But when we gave them a piece of tumor with nothing else, they couldn't tell the difference."

At the time Wolchok posed his question to Bergman, there was a huge and vastly underserved demand for new therapies to treat melanoma in both dogs and people. Each year, about seventy-four thousand new cases of melanoma are diagnosed in Americans, making the disease accountable for 2 percent of all cases of skin cancer in the United States. Nearly ten thousand people are expected to die of the disease each year in the United States alone.[1]

Melanoma accounts for more than 5 percent of skin cancers diagnosed in American dogs, with the most malignant melanomas occurring in the mouth.[2] When Bergman started working with Wolchok, he knew all too well that the prognosis for dogs with melanoma was miserable: those treated with surgery lived on average between three and eighteen months, depending on how advanced the cancer was. Radiation and chemotherapy didn't help much at all.[3]

Wolchok's idea was to trick the immune system into attacking the cancer. His method, called xenogeneic plasmid DNA vaccination, would involve taking DNA from a species other than the one being treated — hence the term xenogeneic — and injecting it into cancer patients. The foreign DNA would be engineered to include a gene that would churn out a "tumor associated antigen" (TAA), which is an abnormal protein produced by tumors. As that protein circulated through the blood, the immune system would recognize it as unwelcome and mount an attack that would kill the melanoma cells.

The TAA Wolchok picked was the protein tyrosinase. Despite its similar-sounding name, tyrosinase is not the same as tyrosine kinase, the protein targeted by Palladia and Sutent. Tyrosinase is a perfectly normal protein that's found in everyone's skin cells and is primarily responsible for creating pigment. Dogs, mice, and other animals have tyrosinase, too, in their mouths and also in their fur follicles, where the protein's main job is to determine what type of coat they will have. But when tyrosinase production grows out of control, melanoma often emerges.

By the time he met Bergman, Wolchok had already completed trials in which he gave human tyrosinase to mice that had been engineered to have melanoma tumors. Their immune systems reacted by attacking the tumors.

"We're only 15 percent different [genetically] from mice," Wolchok explained when I met him to learn more about his vaccine. "But that difference is enough for the immune system to see the protein as being foreign and to react to it. And because we're 85 percent identical, the tools the immune system uses are able to recognize mouse and human equally well. So you vaccinate a mouse with the human target, it recognizes it as being foreign, and it has an immune reaction that can reject melanoma."

Wolchok figured that if he gave human tyrosinase to dogs who had developed melanoma naturally, their immune systems would react by eliminating the melanoma, just as it had done in the mouse models.

When Wolchok explained it to him, Bergman thought the idea was ingenious.

"It basically tries to mimic nature," said Bergman, a tall

man with a football player's build and a quiet demeanor. "Think about it: Our immune system is pre-programmed to react to bacteria, viruses, or anything foreign. So that slight difference between dog and human should be enough to get the dog's immune system to wake up and say, 'Danger! I need to make an immune response to this.'"

Within a few months of meeting at that dinner, Bergman and Wolchok had formulated their vaccine, set up a trial, and recruited nine dogs with melanoma.

The effort to develop cancer vaccines is part of a broader research quest known as cancer immunotherapy. The goal of oncologists working in this field is to treat cancer by capitalizing on the immune system's natural inclination to seize foreign invaders and destroy them.

Vaccines that prevent diseases are usually made of attenuated — weakened — bacteria or viruses that don't cause symptoms themselves, but still prompt the immune system to produce antibodies, which circulate throughout the body. Then, should an actual infectious bacterium or virus invade, the antibodies descend, killing the infection before it starts.

Therapeutic vaccines, such as those being tried in cancer, work on a similar principle, except they eradicate the cancer after it takes hold in the body and continue to prevent recurrences throughout patients' lives. That's the idea, anyway.

The notion that the immune system might be trained to recognize and eliminate cancer has been around since the late 1800s, but it wasn't really taken seriously until the 1960s. That's when a handful of oncologists proposed that the immune system could spot TAAs. But initial efforts to turn that knowledge into some sort of cancer-killing mechanism failed.[4]

In the 1980s, cancer researchers began to better identify and understand TAAs, and the field of cancer immunotherapy was reborn. Many different approaches emerged, but Wolchok's was unusual in its use of DNA from one species to treat a different species.

Despite their having taken different career paths, Bergman and Wolchok made a perfect pair to co-develop the melanoma vaccine. Wolchok, who joined Memorial Sloan Kettering in 1996, had spent his career working in cancer immunotherapy. A slight man with cropped hair and a remarkable ability to multitask, he ran clinical trials for several companies that were developing cancer vaccines, while at the same time treating melanoma patients in his hospital — two demanding tasks that generated three hundred e-mails a day, he told me.

Bergman earned his veterinary degree at Colorado State University, one of the institutes that pioneered comparative oncology research (see Chapter 4), before studying human medicine at MD Anderson. When I spoke to him he had relocated to the Katonah Bedford Veterinary Center in Bedford Hills, New York, where he was assigned to run clinical studies for VCA, a large chain of veterinary clinics, including his. What particularly intrigued him about developing a vaccine for animals using human DNA was that it might ultimately prove useful in other pets that are susceptible to melanoma.

"The xenogeneic premise fits for dogs, cats, horses," Bergman told me.

"Horses get melanoma?" I asked.

They do, he said, though it's driven by a genetic mutation that's not seen in people. The beauty of the vaccine, he explained, was that it would be designed to prompt the immune system to kill all melanomas regardless of whether they were caused by a mutation or something else — even if that something else had yet to be discovered.

———

When Bergman and Wolchok started their dog trial, they were optimistic but not quite sure what to expect. It wasn't long before Bergman found inspiration in an eighty-pound mixed-breed dog who had stage four melanoma that had spread to his chest. When Bergman spoke to the dog's owner, a veterinary technician from Connecticut, he warned her that the melanoma was so advanced, without treatment, her pet would have no more than six weeks to live.

About eight weeks after the dog received the first injection of the experimental vaccine, his tumor stopped growing, Bergman said. One year later, the tumor started to shrink.

"The vaccine was obviously impacting the biology of that patient's disease," Bergman said. "It was unlike anything I had ever seen."

Wolchok had fond memories of a blue-eyed male Siberian husky whose cancer had spread to the lungs. The vaccine gave the husky an additional year of life, far exceeding his or Bergman's expectations.

"For me, that was the beginning of the success," Wolchok said.

But it was the big mutt who was the trial's most surprising survivor. His melanoma vanished completely, along with dozens of other tumors throughout his body. The dog lived melanoma-free for five years before dying of an unrelated cancer — one that was not driven by tyrosinase and therefore would not have responded to the melanoma vaccine.

Two other dogs that were in earlier stages of melanoma when they entered the trial were also cured. The median survival time for all nine dogs in the trial was 389 days, and the only side effect any of them suffered was inflammation of the skin where the vaccine was injected.[5]

From that point on, the two men were on a mission. Their plan was twofold: They wanted to find a company that would help bring their dog vaccine to market. Then they would deploy all the data they had collected from dogs to develop a similar vaccine for use in people. So they hit the road, scheduling pitch meetings with every pharmaceutical company that had an animal health division.

"I distinctly remember all of them saying, 'This won't work. It's too crazy an idea. Go away,'" Bergman said. Even the organizations that provide funding for clinical trials designed to help animals turned them down.

Then in April 2001, the United States Department of Agriculture (USDA) got wind of Bergman and Wolchok's research and invited the two scientists to present their work at a conference — "Biologics for Cancer Diagnosis, Prevention and Immunotherapy" — at Iowa State University in Ames.

Even though the FDA is in charge of approving most drugs to treat cancer in people and animals in the United States, the USDA has jurisdiction over most injectable animal drugs that modulate the immune system. That includes all vaccines, as well as several other "large molecules" — protein-based drugs that work via immune pathways in the body.

Starting with a law passed in the early 1900s — when rapid approvals of new drugs were needed to control massive outbreaks of diseases among livestock, poultry, and other food animals — the USDA put several processes in place to speed new products to market.[6] For example, the agency now could green-light new drugs on a conditional basis, with data from trials involving a small number of animals. Companies that were granted those conditional approvals could go ahead and sell their new products while simultaneously completing larger studies necessary to get the full license.

But USDA officials had no experience approving cancer therapeutics for pets, so they convened the Iowa conference to gather more information about the drugs coming down the pipeline. For the two young researchers from New York City, the experience of presenting their research to the USDA was unforgettable.

"There we were, driving up the highway from Des Moines to Ames, with cornfields on one side and pig farms on the other," Wolchok said. "Being from New York, this was a very interesting introduction to the deep Midwest. We gave our presentation, and we got a lot of positive feedback."

One woman sitting in the front row was particularly interested in the cancer vaccine they had developed, Wolchok recalled. Her name was Louise Henderson, and she was the USDA official in charge of policy evaluation and product licensing. She told Bergman and Wolchok that she believed their vaccine was promising, but that they had violated two federal statutes in doing that first trial, first by shipping the vaccine from Wolchok's lab to the Animal Medical Center, and then by failing to inform the New York state veterinarian that they were doing a clinical trial.

Wolchok was mortified to learn he might have broken the law.

"I was feeling rather cheeky at the time," he told me, "and I said, 'Oh, but Dr. Henderson, we didn't have to ship it. I walked the vaccine down the street.'"

Henderson informed Wolchok that the moment he walked out the door of the facility where the vaccine was made, with the product in his hand, he was actually shipping it. Feeling a bit sheepish, Wolchok and Bergman stepped off the stage, and Wolchok whispered a question about the second statute the two had apparently violated.

"I said to Phil, 'Is there a state veterinarian?' And he said, 'Every state has a veterinarian.'"

The two men were relieved when it took only a day or so to get both the shipping authorization and their trial approved by the state veterinarian.

"Generally the USDA is not going to take action against somebody — they're going to educate somebody," Henderson told me when I reached her by phone to get her take on the Ames meeting. "The USDA is charged with

63

protecting animals. We wanted to keep an objective eye on the product but also have the chance to say, 'Yes, you can move forward.'"

Also in the audience that day were scientists from the veterinary products maker Merial, which was at the time a joint venture of pharmaceutical giants Merck and Sanofi-Aventis. The Merial employees invited Wolchok and Bergman to their offices in New Jersey to tell them more about the melanoma vaccine.

The two researchers weren't optimistic they'd get a fair hearing at Merial, Wolchok recalled, especially since the company was in the process of moving from New Jersey to Georgia. But they went in the hopes that Merial would agree to further develop the vaccine, and in a room full of packed boxes, they stood up and presented their data to the small group that had come to hear them.

The reaction of the Merial scientists was quite different from any the oncologist and veterinarian had heard before. The company's researchers thought they could bring valuable input to the project, as they had developed and successfully marketed several vaccines to prevent infectious diseases in cats, dogs, and livestock. They were game to move the therapeutic vaccine forward, even though there was no precedent to indicate whether pet owners and veterinarians would embrace the product.

"The market for cancer therapeutics is much smaller than the infectious disease markets," said Tim Leard, senior research and development leader for vaccines and biotherapeutics at Merial, when I discussed the project with him.

But Leard had been a practicing veterinarian for twelve

years before joining the pharmaceutical industry, and the memories of all the hopeless melanoma cases he had treated were still on his mind. "We didn't expect to be able to create silver bullets, but anything we could do to prolong survival times for these patients would be a good thing," he said.

Merial took over the project, providing the funding for a second, larger trial, and lending the vaccine's two inventors the expertise they needed to navigate the regulatory process. In 2007, thanks to the USDA's expedited review process, Merial won permission to sell the drug — which was later named Oncept — while it was completing the larger trial.

For that crucial trial, fifty-eight dogs with stage two or three oral melanoma were treated with the vaccine for six months at five veterinary clinics around the country. Rather than comparing those dogs to traditional controls — dogs with melanoma who would be treated with a placebo or perhaps chemotherapy — the researchers used historical controls. These were dogs who had been treated in past clinical trials with placebos or who had been given drugs that had little measurable impact on their melanoma.

Henderson, who had left the USDA in 2008 to work as a private consultant to developers of veterinary products, told me that the ability to assess new products based on historical controls was particularly important for drugs being developed to treat companion animals. That's because it's difficult for veterinarians to recruit pet owners for trials when they have to tell some of them that their cats or dogs might get a placebo or something else that's unlikely to work.

"Those animals clearly are individually important to their owners — we're not talking about a herd or a flock situation," Henderson said. "It's important for researchers to be able to prove the product works, but we wanted them to be able to do that in a manner that didn't introduce more heartache."

After Merial took over the development of Oncept, Bergman continued to study the drug on his own, offering it to clients who had no other options and observing their dogs' responses for more clues about where the product might best be used. Among the dogs to participate in that research was Puccini, a thirteen-year-old cocker spaniel owned by Manhattan real estate executive Linda Wassong. In May 2006, Wassong noticed a bump under Puccini's right eye. Thinking it was an abscessed tooth, she took the dog to a local veterinary dentist. A few hours later, Wassong was getting her hair dyed at a beauty salon when her phone rang.

"The vet said, 'I'm sorry, your dog has melanoma,'" Wassong recalled. Devastated, she ran out of the salon with her hair still wet, jumped in a cab, and ran to get Puccini.

"You're not supposed to cry in front of [dogs], because they'll know something is wrong. So there I was, all chipper in that car. But all I kept thinking was, 'My dog has melanoma and he's going to die,'" she said.

Wassong took Puccini to his regular veterinarian, who told her about Bergman's trial, which had recently started. She immediately called the Animal Medical Center and applied to get Puccini into the trial, even though she had never heard of a melanoma vaccine before and didn't quite grasp how it was meant to work.

The world is rife with tear-inducing dog stories, but when I sat down with Wassong to hear Puccini's story years later, I realized that this was more than a typical woman-loves-dog tale. Wassong found Puccini as a puppy, when on a whim she walked into a pet store to play with some pugs she saw in the window. The cocker spaniel stared at her until she played with him, too. Afterward, she couldn't get the spaniel out of her mind, so that Friday, after work, she bought the dog and brought him home.

Puccini got his name that first night, while Wassong was listening to the composer's opera *Turandot*. But the dog's presence wasn't quite as calming as his namesake's music.

"That whole weekend, Puccini kept mounting me — my arm, my leg, my finger, my face," Wassong said, laughing at the memory.

After the local vet diagnosed Puccini with a dominance problem, Wassong tried to crate train the dog, but that only made matters worse.

"When he got into a crate, he would turn it upside down and all the nuts and bolts would fall out," she told me.

Puccini was so food-obsessed he would jump on the table or the kitchen counter, as if he were a cat, and eat whatever he found. He was loyal and loving with Wassong, but whenever visitors came over, he barked incessantly at them and invariably tried to mount them. Wassong tried all the well-known remedies, like shaking a can of coins at him every time he barked, but he wouldn't stop.

"He just did what he wanted," she said.

Wassong hired the renowned dog trainer Bash Dibra, but even he couldn't figure out how to tame Puccini. Dibra told Wassong the dog's problems likely stemmed from having been born in a puppy mill, and he urged her to return the dog to the pet store. She refused.

When Puccini was about eight, Wassong decided a canine companion might be the key to easing his anxieties. So she adopted another cocker spaniel, named Sparkle. The two dogs became inseparable.

Wassong spent summers on Long Island, where she often drove a Jeep onto the beach, unleashed the dogs, and let them sprint up and down the shore. It was after one of those jaunts that Wassong first noticed the melanoma.

Wassong was elated when Puccini was accepted into the vaccine trial. She packed up the dog, along with Sparkle, and went straight to Bergman's office, where he carefully explained how the vaccine worked and what the treatment plan would be: Puccini would get the vaccine, then four booster shots, and a chest x-ray six months later to make sure the cancer wasn't spreading. When he told Wassong the trial might help people too, she was sold.

"I realized Puccini had an opportunity to do something incredible," Wassong said. "Everybody facing cancer has their hope moment, whatever 'hope' means to them. I walked out of there and I had my hope moment."

For the next six months, Wassong said, Puccini was his old self, stealing food, running along the beach, never acting sick. But when Bergman x-rayed his lungs at the dog's first follow-up appointment, he found the cancer had spread. There were no treatments left to try, so Wassong kept the dog comfortable for as long as she could, finally making the decision to have him euthanized a few months later. During her last weeks with Puccini, she vowed to find a way to support the researchers who had tried to save his life.

"I promised Puccini I would do something to create awareness of comparative oncology," Wassong said. "I think this is amazing science."

Of the fifty-eight dogs who received the melanoma vaccine in Merial's trial, fewer than half died from their disease before the end of the designated trial period, so the researchers were unable to compute the median survival time for the entire group.[7] To them this seemed like a good problem, though they knew the veterinarians they'd be counting on to prescribe the vaccine might not agree.

"Oncologists are always looking for data — they live for this 'median survival time,'" said Robert Menardi, Merial's director of veterinary technical solutions. "In some ways, we had to fight the absence of the number, even though the absence of the number was a very positive thing."

Indeed, as the company reported in the published trial, eight of the dogs were still alive with no signs of cancer when the researchers were wrapping up their analysis. Another sixteen had died of causes unrelated to melanoma.[8]

Those unrelated deaths were the only ones that worried Wolchok. Two of the dogs were being treated during the summer at a veterinary clinic in Texas. They drowned accidentally when they were out with their owners for a swim. There's little chance the drownings were related to the drug, Wolchok said, but had just one more dog suffered the same unfortunate fate, the researchers might have been required to slap a warning label on the drug saying it might cause drowning.

"If enough of these events pile up that statistically raise concerns about an unforeseen side effect, that becomes part of the safety profile of the medicine," Wolchok said. "But it was just bad luck."

In the end, the USDA was satisfied that the drug worked and was safe to roll out to veterinary clinics around the country. The agency granted Oncept a full license in February 2010, making it the first ever therapeutic vaccine approved to treat cancer — in either animals or people.[9]

Wolchok and his colleagues at Memorial Sloan Kettering wanted to try a similar approach in people. But they couldn't use the same vaccine that had been given to dogs because it contained human DNA — and to fool the immune system they needed to use DNA from a different species than that being treated. So they chose to test a human vaccine made with mouse DNA instead.

To observe the immune response, they took eighteen patients with late-stage melanoma and divided them into two groups. The first group received the mouse-based vaccine, followed by injections of human DNA (similar to what the dogs got). The second group got the same vaccines, but in the opposite sequence. Wolchok explained that his team used both mouse and human DNA vaccines in the trials because they had seen early evidence during the rodent trials that starting with the foreign gene and then switching to the endogenous gene boosted the immune response. Wolchok and his colleagues assessed the response by measuring the patients' T cells, which are crucial players in the body's immune response. They found that some of the patients showed signs of a positive immune response regardless of whether they got the mouse DNA first or second.[10]

Unfortunately, the response wasn't potent enough to merit pursuing the xenogeneic vaccine approach in people any further, Wolchok said. During the dog and human trials, his team uncovered some key characteristics of the biology of the human immune system that they came to believe were the reason for the muted response in people. I wondered if the discovery disappointed him. On the contrary, Wolchok told me. He believed the Oncept trials had helped guide the entire field of immunotherapy.

"There had never been a clinical trial in any species that delivered the degree of positive efficacy data that these [dog] studies did," Wolchok said. "This provided a meaningful benchmark of success."

———

Bergman's VCA clinic in Westchester County, New York, is situated on a main street in the affluent town of Bedford Hills. It employs nearly twenty vets, whose specialties include dentistry, alternative medicine, nutrition, neurology, and cardiology. I visited Bergman on a busy summer day, when the waiting room was full.

Among the visitors that day were a thirteen-year-old beagle named Heathcliff and his owner, Kim Catania, who adopted him as a puppy. Heathcliff had been on Oncept for almost a year. The aggressive, gumball-sized melanoma that had been removed from his mouth showed no signs of returning, Catania told me, as Heathcliff ambled around Bergman's office, panting and lapping water from the bowl the veterinarian placed on the floor for him.

Catania, a pharmaceutical industry consultant, hadn't heard of the vaccine before Bergman recommended it for Heathcliff, but she was fascinated by the technology and the goal of developing a similar product for people. With her background in drug development, she had a few more questions for Bergman than the average dog owner would have had.

"He explained everything," said Catania. "We discussed the risks and benefits, and even though [Heathcliff] was older, I thought it would be worth it because his Q of L would be good."

"Q of L" is pharma industry jargon for quality of life, and it is one of the main factors that's taken into account by patients and dog owners when deciding whether to pursue radical but potentially life-saving cancer treatments. For Catania, maintaining Heathcliff's Q of L meant ensuring he could still enjoy dashing around their two-and-a-half-acre yard, howling at squirrels and birds, or teasing her two other dogs, a beagle–German short-haired pointer mix and a Labrador retriever.

Catania said she often referred to Heathcliff as the Jan Brady of the house — a reference to the 1970s TV hit *The Brady Bunch* about a blended family — because he was so independent that whenever she curled up on the couch with her other dogs, Heathcliff wouldn't join them; he'd plop himself on the other side of the room. The only sign of his cancer battle was a faded scar on his face where the tumor had been. The scar pulled the side of his mouth into a faint sneer that befitted his slightly cantankerous nature.

The plan for Heathcliff was to continue giving him booster shots of Oncept every six months for as long as he remained healthy, Bergman said. The beagle was one of the many success stories he was quickly racking up for Oncept.

Bergman was particularly excited that day, because he had started to receive e-mails from horse owners thanking him for inventing Oncept. He learned that cases of melanoma had been proliferating in aged gray mares, and preliminary research at the University of Tennessee had shown the dog vaccine to be safe and effective in horses with the disease.[11]

"Heathcliff was a perfect example of using the drug on label — for what it's approved to do," Bergman said. "But we know that whether it's a dog, a cat, or a person, melanoma over-expresses the antigen of interest, tyrosinase. So it makes sense that it would potentially have efficacy in other situations. So we're now getting lots of really cool e-mails from owners across the country about how well their horses are responding to the vaccine."

Bergman regaled us with stories about his other patients who had done well on Oncept. There was Nellie, a twelve-year-old black pug who had been on the drug for two years, and was still successfully fending off the aggressive oral melanoma that had threatened her life. And there was Stripie, a regal-looking black-and-brown striped cat who was on Oncept for three years before he died of kidney failure at age fourteen, cancer-free.

But the dog that most amazed Bergman was a miniature schnauzer named Sunny Boy. The dog, owned by a Connecticut family, had developed a melanoma behind his eye when he was six years old. The eye was removed and the dog seemed fine until three years later, when a tumor showed up in his liver. Kathy Novak, Sunny Boy's owner, was referred to Bergman.

The veterinarian had heard about people who developed melanomas in their eyes and were successfully treated, only to end up with melanoma in their livers ten or fifteen or even twenty years later. Sunny Boy was facing exactly the same scenario.

"Never in my career had I seen this syndrome in dogs," Bergman said. "There's some predisposition in the melanoma cells that causes them to be quiescent for decades and then to metastasize. We don't understand the mechanism."

Nor was there any precedent in people or dogs to help him decide whether the melanoma vaccine would help Sunny Boy. Bergman and Novak decided to try it anyway.

Three years later, Novak told me, Sunny Boy was cancer-free, taking long walks and sniffing every corner, as his breed — which was originally developed to catch rats — was famous for doing. The vaccine booster cost $600 every six months, and Sunny Boy had had to have part of his liver removed, which cost nearly $8,000. But Novak had no regrets. The family's desire to save the dog brought them to the Magic Bullet Fund, a Connecticut-based non-profit that provided financial assistance to people whose dogs were being treated for cancer. The fund kicked in $2,500 for Sunny Boy's treatments.

"As long as we had a good, fighting chance, we were going to find a way to do it," Novak said. "We're still paying it off to this day. Some people might say it's crazy to spend that much on a pet, but we really love our dog."

Bergman and Wolchok believed the Oncept approach would work in other animal cancers, such as lymphoma and osteosarcoma. Bergman's goal was to develop vaccines for those diseases, but instead of inserting the gene for tyrosinase, he intended to use antigens specific to lymphoma and osteosarcoma and the genes that make those antigens instead. He also wanted to develop a vaccine against feline mammary tumors that expressed HER2, a genetic mutation that's linked to many cases of breast cancer in women, too.

"The beauty of that technology is that the DNA can stay the same except for one little piece that's inserted," Bergman said.

Wolchok was also excited about the future of xenogeneic vaccines for treating cancer in animals. He was working with Bergman to examine the potential of developing a lymphoma vaccine containing human DNA and a mammary cancer vaccine containing rat DNA.

Tim Leard couldn't tell me exactly what Merial had planned in building upon its Oncept franchise, except to say he was confident the xenogeneic approach could be applied to other cancers.

"We have a fairly powerful proof-of-concept with our initial product," he said.

Wolchok's contribution to the field of cancer immunotherapy reached far beyond his work on Oncept. He led key clinical trials for ipilimumab (later given the trade name Yervoy), a drug that targeted a group of immune cells called cytotoxic T lymphocytes. These lymphocytes naturally recognize and destroy cancer cells in people but sometimes get turned off in patients with melanoma. The drug was designed to reactivate the cells. Its approval in 2011 was hailed by many as the beginning of a new era of immunotherapy in cancer, and within two years it was bringing in nearly $1 billion a year for its manufacturer, Bristol-Myers Squibb.

On October 28, 2013, Bergman and Wolchok were honored for their contributions to cancer immunotherapy at a celebration held at the Griffis Faculty Club at New York Presbyterian Hospital and sponsored by the Puccini Foundation, the non-profit that Linda Wassong started in memory of the cocker spaniel she lost to melanoma. Her goal was to raise money and awareness for comparative oncology, and this was her first big splash.

The club was decked out with photos of many of the dogs who had been treated with Oncept at Bergman's clinic, and wine coasters featured a photo of Wassong's beloved Puccini. An opera singer, accompanied by a small group of chamber musicians, sang the composer's famous arias as Wassong made the rounds, thanking everyone who had contributed to her new foundation.

Just before the awards ceremony started, I ran into Kathy Novak. I asked her how Sunny Boy was feeling.

"He's eleven and a half now," she told me. "He has no symptoms."

Bergman was the first to be called up to receive his award. As he turned to face the crowd, he smiled, and tears began to roll down his face.

"Many of my clients are here — people who brought their pets to me and had this crazy idea to try a vaccine," he said, apologizing to the crowd for his emotional response to the honor.

Wolchok told me he wasn't surprised by his friend's tears. Much of the reason he and Bergman hit it off in the first place, he said, was that they were both as dedicated to taking good care of their patients as they were to oncology research.

"We were both considered young investigators, both trained at prominent institutions — we had every reason to be egomaniacal. But that was not part of his DNA, nor mine," Wolchok said. "We saw in each other the perfect counterpart. We were not in this to make a name for ourselves. We're still not. We are committed to the bigger goal of helping patients and advancing science. The outpouring of recognition and appreciation is strong, strong motivation to work harder."

Chapter 4
Burying Bone Cancer

Emily Brown was eleven years old when, in early 1997, a bone tumor the size of a grapefruit collapsed her spinal cord and left her paralyzed from the waist down. Physicians at Denver Children's Hospital diagnosed her with osteosarcoma of the spine. The vivacious blonde girl, a tomboy who loved roller-skating with her older brother near their home in Colorado Springs and playing with the family's golden retriever, endured ten months of chemotherapy and radiation, and an eighteen-hour marathon surgery that involved removing the tumor, along with four ribs, some vertebrae, and part of her left lung. To boost its potency, her doctors included in her chemo an experimental protein-based drug that was developed, in part, by veterinarians and that had shown great promise in dogs with the same type of bone cancer that Emily had.

That October, Emily's physicians at Denver Children's Hospital discovered that despite everything they had done, there was a mass near her lungs — a likely sign her cancer had progressed. They told her parents, Jeanette and Allyn, that their daughter had three months to live. Emily decided to stop all treatment and put her life on fast forward, so she could experience all the milestones she believed she would never see. She celebrated a mock prom and twenty-first birthday with her family, and realized her Make-a-Wish fantasy of visiting Disney World.

But the Browns were puzzled by what wasn't happening: Emily wasn't in excruciating pain, as her doctors had predicted she would be by her third month off therapy. She barely felt sick at all.

In February 1998, Emily returned to the hospital for exploratory surgery. Her doctors were stunned to discover that there was no sign of cancer. The mass they had seen was merely an inflammation, which they chalked up to an allergic response to a patch they had placed along her spinal cord to protect it.

To keep her cancer from returning, Emily's doctors put her back on the experimental chemo regimen, which she continued until May 1998. She went on to graduate from high school and college, and when I spoke to her in 2013, she was twenty-eight, cancer-free, and helping to manage her cousin's electrical contracting business. Even though her treatments stunted her growth, she had grown to a respectable five foot four and had regained complete use of her legs. Every year on October 22 — the anniversary of the day she was told she was dying — Emily celebrated "Glad to Be Alive Day," during which she wrote a letter to her friends and family detailing all the previous year's experiences she once believed she would never have.

"I'd spent three months basically dying," Emily told me. "But I wasn't dying. It was shocking."

———

Osteosarcoma is a rare but devastating disease that strikes about eight hundred people a year in the United States — half of them children.[1] It's the form of cancer that Terry Fox lost his leg to before he set out in 1980 on his famous attempt to run across Canada, raising money for cancer research. For decades, oncologists who treated osteosarcoma had no choice but to amputate the cancerous limbs.

The development of advanced chemotherapy techniques boosted the five-year survival rate for osteosarcoma patients under the age of fifteen from 40 percent in the 1970s to 68 percent by 1990.[2] But for patients with metastatic disease, the outlook was still grim, and for children like Emily whose tumors were not in their limbs, amputation was not an option.

Osteosarcoma is far more prevalent in dogs, primarily striking large breeds like Great Danes, Saint Bernards, and golden retrievers at a rate of about eight thousand every year in the United States.[3] More than a half-dozen genes implicated in the human pediatric form of the cancer have also been found in the canine version,[4] which is why osteosarcoma is considered a prime candidate for comparative studies.

Emily believes she owes her life to a drug that was originally tested in dogs, muramyl tripeptide phosphatidylethanolamine (MTP-PE). She received the drug after she was accepted into a clinical trial, in which 677 osteosarcoma patients were randomly assigned to receive one of four treatment regimens, two of which included MTP-PE. Emily's treatment consisted of MTP-PE as part of a chemo cocktail that also included doxorubicin, methotrexate, ifosfamide, and cisplatin.

MTP-PE works by targeting macrophages, which are white blood cells in the immune system that devour pathogens and mobilize other immune cells to fight illnesses. The veterinarians investigating MTP-PE in the original trials wanted to prove that when added to chemotherapy, the drug would essentially reprogram macrophages, making them home in on cancer cells and destroy them.

How Emily's oncologists found out about MTP-PE is a tale of cross-collaboration — across hospitals, medical specialties, and even species. Emily's primary physician, Lia Gore, was completing her fellowship at Denver Children's Hospital when she learned that MTP-PE would be tested in a trial sponsored by the Children's Oncology Group, an international consortium of two hundred children's hospitals, including Denver's. Gore had heard from Stephen J. Withrow, a veterinarian and professor who worked at Colorado State University in Fort Collins, that MTP-PE had worked well in dogs. Oncologists at Denver Children's often tapped Withrow for advice, because they knew some of the newest ideas for treating cancer in kids were being pioneered by the people who were curing the disease in dogs.

"The biology of osteosarcoma in a Labrador retriever is the same as it is in a five-year-old or a forty-year-old," Gore said. "Obviously, I'm not going to treat the Labrador and Steve Withrow isn't going to treat the five-year-old, but we do a lot of crosstalk. Steve and I were trading e-mails three or four times a month at a minimum, and sometimes three or four times an hour."

Gore learned that in 1995, a team at the University of Wisconsin led by veterinarian E. Gregory MacEwen had achieved the longest median survival time ever reported in dogs with osteosarcoma, thanks to MTP-PE. During two studies, dogs whose diseased limbs were amputated subsequently received either chemotherapy with MTP-PE or chemo alone. The MTP-PE extended survival from 9.8 months to 14.4 months. Sixteen of the fifty-three dogs who received MTP-PE during the trials lived for more than a year longer. Four were cured. Some dogs in the trial developed fevers, but for the most part, their owners could easily manage the side effects.[5]

That research gave Gore the evidence she needed to persuade Emily's parents to enter their daughter into the human trials of MTP-PE.

"I was able to say, 'This looks really promising in animal models. It increases the immune system's ability to scavenge for cancer cells in the lungs,'" Gore said.

Jeanette and Allyn Brown agreed to the trial, knowing that, even if Emily's participation didn't extend her life, it would most definitely contribute to the understanding of a novel therapy that could help children in the future.

Gore and the rest of Emily's treatment team could never fully explain why their young patient's cancer disappeared. They suspected the immune response that MTP-PE produced persisted beyond the period in which the drug was actually administered. So even during the few months when Emily was off all her medications, it's possible her macrophages were still launching raids against any cancer cells that emerged.

"That was the only drug that could, in any way, shape, or form, still have been working in that time period," Emily said. "I believe that's what ultimately made those tumors go away."

The choice to participate in the trial did not come without costs, though. Emily developed such a high fever after her first treatment that she had to be re-admitted to the hospital. After that, she was pre-treated with anti-inflammatories before each dose. The five-drug assault left Emily with a litany of permanent health problems — hearing loss, restricted breathing, kidney damage. She got so sick during her freshman year at Vanderbilt University in Nashville that Jeanette had to move into her dorm room to help her get through the semester. Emily ended up transferring to the University of Colorado so she could live at home. Still, she has never regretted undergoing the experimental treatment.

"Was it bad? Beyond compare," she said. "But now, sixteen years later, I don't remember a lot of it. The bad never outweighed the good."

In 2005, the Children's Oncology Group published the results of the MTP-PE trial. They reported that adding the protein to the four-drug chemo regimen boosted the probability of survival at five years from 53 percent to 72 percent. Emily was counted among the survivors.[6]

MTP-PE isn't the only osteosarcoma innovation championed by Withrow that helped Emily. After her surgeons removed part of her diseased spine, they replaced it with bone grafts in a procedure similar to one that Withrow developed in the 1980s for dogs with osteosarcoma.

The term "comparative oncology" didn't exist back then, and there was virtually no dialogue between veterinarians and physicians. But Withrow wanted to help children and dogs with bone cancer. So he figured out how to remove the tumors from dogs with osteosarcoma and replace the bone with grafts made from the donated bones of deceased pets.

Then Withrow took it upon himself to share his idea with surgeons who treated people. Oncologists slowly began to adopt the technique, called "limb sparing," and by the end of the 1990s it was the treatment of choice.

With the help of their canine patients, Withrow and his team of veterinarians tested all sorts of new ideas for combating bone cancer. They developed new ways of delivering chemotherapy, and they perfected bone grafts by making them with advanced synthetic materials that rendered the repaired limbs more durable. Any veterinarian around the world with a new idea for combating bone cancer invariably turned to the scientists at CSU to help test it.

I asked Emily if learning how dogs had contributed to her cure made her look any differently at her own pets. She told me that she was born into a family of golden retriever lovers, and when she looked in the eyes of her four-year-old golden, Gertrude Chubbs, she couldn't help but think about how dogs might help scientists develop better, less toxic cures for kids with cancer.

"Dogs have always been part of our family, but even more so now," she said. "I truly believe they are pathways to understanding all cancer."

———

CSU's Flint Animal Cancer Center is nestled in a residential neighborhood two miles south of the main campus in Fort Collins, a town of 151,000. A bronze statue of a playful foal greeting a cat marks the entrance of the veterinary school's sprawling campus, which encompasses the small-animal clinic, the cancer center, and the large-animal hospital. More than thirty thousand animals are treated at CSU's vet school every year[7] — including about fifteen hundred dogs and cats that have been newly diagnosed with cancer.[8]

Each day at the oncology center starts with rounds, a meeting of about twenty staff vets and students, who trade notes on all of the patients scheduled to be seen that day. When I visited CSU to meet Withrow and learn more about his pioneering work, I started my day by sitting in on rounds.

In the rounds room, all the ongoing trials were listed on a whiteboard, categorized by disease: osteosarcoma, mast cell tumors, lymphoma. One by one, the veterinarians updated everyone on the pets they were treating, starting with the dogs. One vet brought up the case of a twelve-year-old Lab named Jake, who was suffering from soft-tissue sarcoma that had started in his leg and metastasized to his lungs. Jake had already undergone a partial amputation.

"Jake has told his owner he doesn't want chemo," the vet said. A few quiet chuckles rippled around the room. "It sounds cuckoo," the vet acknowledged, "but if you met this woman, you'd be amazed at the insight she has into her dog."

The conversation was a reflection of one of CSU's biggest priorities — teaching veterinary students the importance of compassion. The veterinary hospital is home to the Argus Institute, a group of full-time counselors who work with grieving pet owners, and also with veterinarians to teach them how to provide emotional support to clients facing tough decisions, such as whether to try experimental treatments or to euthanize their pets.

Argus organizes seminars for veterinary students, hiring actors to dramatize the range of anxious scenarios that play out every day in the clinic, and critiquing the students' responses. One actor might play a client angry about an enormous bill, while another might portray a baffled and devastated dog owner trying to understand a cancer diagnosis.

"It's about learning how to listen," Withrow told me after rounds, when I sat down to talk with him in his office.

Withrow literally wrote the book on treating cancer in pets — the textbook *Small Animal Clinical Oncology*, part of the canon at vet schools worldwide — which he co-authored in 1989 with Greg MacEwen (who died in 2001). Withrow retired from CSU in May 2012, but he held on to his office at the veterinary cancer center and still spent most of his time there. The fifth edition of his textbook was published a few months after his retirement, and several boxes of the book were stacked on the floor of his office.

Withrow told me he kept busy in his retirement recruiting donors for a $30 million expansion of the cancer center, which was originally built in 2002. He pointed out his window at a large plot of vacant land that he told potential donors would be a cancer innovation center. The center would provide more space for veterinarians and scientists to work together on comparative projects.

Withrow had a gift for making friends with big-name animal lovers: Among the donors who helped build CSU's presence in veterinary oncology were Elbridge Hadley Stuart, a member of the Carnation Milk family dynasty; General Norman Schwarzkopf; and famed Weimaraner photographer William Wegman, whose dog Fay Ray came to CSU to be treated for leukemia. The cancer center was named for ink industry magnate Robert H. Flint and his wife, Mary. They donated $3 million toward its construction in memory of their two Labrador retrievers, both of whom were treated for cancer at CSU.[9]

Withrow got into bone cancer as his specialty by chance in 1975, when he was a newly minted veterinarian learning the human side of medicine during a fellowship at the Mayo Clinic in Rochester, Minnesota. Withrow, a native Minnesotan, joined the hospital's hockey team, which was mostly made up of orthopedic oncologists. It was not long after Edward "Ted" Kennedy Jr., then age twelve, lost a leg to osteosarcoma. During practices and games, the team often commiserated about the dire prognosis for children facing the disease.

After Withrow joined CSU in 1978 as a junior faculty member, he began investigating a concept called downstaging.

"One technique we developed on pet dogs was to take this big, bad, nasty tumor and convert it into a small tumor," he said. They did it by pre-treating the patient with chemotherapy, rather than following the standard practice of surgery first, chemo second. Shrinking the tumor first made it more feasible to remove it without having to amputate the entire limb. Downstaging eventually became standard practice among pediatricians treating osteosarcoma, he said.

From there, Withrow began investigating materials that could be used to replace cancerous bone with functional, healthy tissue. In 1984, he met Ross Wilkins, an orthopedic oncologist in Denver, who decided then and there he wanted to join the quest to develop better osteosarcoma treatments.

"When I started in this business, it was absolutely terrible," Wilkins told me. "I'd biopsy these ten-year-old kids, find out they had bone cancer, quickly do an amputation, and then literally wait for them to die. One of my crusades with Steve was that we just had to find a better way. So we started looking at dogs — what worked, what didn't work — and talking with other [oncologists] around the country who had experience on the human side."

Wilkins and Withrow brainstormed solutions to the variety of problems they encountered, including the high rate of infection among patients receiving donor bones.

"Early on we'd put these big pieces of donor bone in

dogs or people and we'd get problems," Wilkins said. "It wouldn't heal, or, because it was foreign, it would get infected. Or, the body would accept it but then start dissolving it away, so it would break."

One night over pizza, Wilkins and Withrow began scribbling ideas on a paper napkin, among them taking all the marrow out of the center of the donor bone and replacing it with bone cement made from a type of acrylic. Then they figured they should add an antibiotic to the cement, so the medicine would leech into the bone and prevent infection. They perfected the technique, called cement-augmented cortical autograft, in the laboratory. Then Withrow tried it in his canine patients and found that bone grafts containing the cement healed as well as or better than traditional bone grafts, fractures were nearly eliminated, and infection rates went down.

Wilkins tried the technique in his pediatric patients. Again, it worked.

"That technique is used worldwide now, and it has decreased the complication rate by about 30 percent," Wilkins said. "This relationship with CSU — this bond between dogs and kids who get the same bone cancer — it's good for healing."

Veterinarian Rodney Page, who took over the directorship of CSU's animal cancer center after Withrow retired, was taking me on a tour of the veterinary cancer clinic when we were nearly knocked to the ground by a drooling Saint

Bernard and a giant black-and-white mixed-breed dog. The two were patients, Page explained, who were waiting in line to receive a treatment called stereotactic radiation therapy (SRT). A third patient, a Rottweiler, was asleep on a table and was being positioned by a team of veterinarians to receive the treatment.

SRT, which is often called gamma knife radiation, is now commonplace in human medicine, but CSU is among only a small handful of veterinary centers offering the therapy, Page explained. SRT uses a room-sized machine called a linear accelerator to focus a powerful beam of radiation on a tumor with a degree of precision that equals that of a surgeon wielding a scalpel. It's used to shrink tumors — to relieve pain, to eradicate the cancer, or ideally both. CSU was studying the technique in dogs to see if it might someday replace surgery altogether.

The biggest challenge of SRT was not in the treatment itself, but rather in positioning the dog in the machine correctly, so the radiation beam would hit the tumor without damaging the surrounding tissue. Page showed me a collection of molds that were made to fit specific dogs and hold them in place during the procedure. Pets receiving SRT had to be anesthetized, he explained, so they wouldn't wriggle around while they were being treated.

Colorado's veterinary school trains students in more than fifteen specialties, including dermatology, equine orthopedics, and zoological medicine, but it is best known for its oncology center — the largest in the world. It draws the interest of the most prominent names in cancer research. Page said he had been working to strengthen ties with institutions that had approached CSU with ideas for comparative oncology projects, including the Mayo Clinic in Scottsdale, Arizona, the MD Anderson Cancer Center in Houston, and the American Society of Clinical Oncology, which is one of the largest networks of cancer physicians, with thirty-five thousand members worldwide.

Page said one of his goals in expanding the center was to provide space for veterinary scientists to work on projects alongside researchers from the main campus who were studying human biology and medicine.

"CSU has some basic science faculty studying biochemistry, structural biology, and everything else related to what makes a cancer cell different," Page said. "This is research that really crosses species. The university recognizes that opportunity."

As we walked down the long hallway away from the linear accelerator, Page pointed out two laboratories staffed by scientists who were entirely focused on studying bone cancer. Despite all the advancements in treating the disease over the years, Page said, there were still many problems left to solve.

Osteosarcoma is particularly vexing because it has a tendency to spread, even after the primary tumor or even the entire diseased limb is removed. One of CSU's priorities was to help develop drugs that could bolster the immune system's ability to recognize these wayward cancer cells and eradicate them before they could travel away from the original tumor site.

In 2008, CSU joined a study led by veterinarians at the University of Minnesota, who wanted to test a form of gene therapy in dogs with osteosarcoma. The treatment consisted of a modified virus molecule, or "vector," which carried a therapeutic gene directly to the tumor site. Once in place at the tumor, the gene churned out a protein called Fas ligand (FasL for short), which had proven in some rodent studies to be a powerful anti-cancer agent.[10]

FasL binds to the surface of tumor cells and prompts them, in essence, to commit suicide. This process, called apoptosis or programmed cell death, occurs naturally in all the cells of the body. Oncology researchers around the world were looking for drugs that could activate apoptosis inside tumors, so metastasizing cells would self-destruct. FasL was considered one of the most promising candidates.

The problem, in rodent studies, was that targeting FasL produced mixed results — it shrank tumors in some cases while encouraging them to grow and spread in others.[11] To understand what FasL was doing in the body, the Minnesota-led team turned to pet dogs.

Their plan was to treat the tumors with gene therapy plus chemo, then track the time to metastasis compared to that in dogs who received chemo alone. To get a closer look at what was happening on a molecular level, they first removed the cancerous limbs. In dogs, amputation was still the preferred treatment for osteosarcoma — it immediately relieved the cancerous pain, and dogs adapted well to living with three legs.

A black Labrador retriever named Emmy was among the first to be enrolled in the gene therapy trial. Emmy was owned by veterinary technician Kathi Streeter and her veterinarian husband, Ron, who live in Franktown,

Colorado, about one hundred miles from csu's campus.

I visited the Streeters, who live on a small ranch with one horse, two barn cats, two canaries, and three rambunctious black Labs. I parked under a tree in the front yard, and one of the dogs, her fur streaked with gray, scurried up to the driver's side door to greet me. She escorted me to the front door, smiling and panting as she trotted beside me.

"That's Ruby," Kathi said as she opened the door and showed me into the kitchen. "Ruby is Emmy's sister from a different litter. We liked Emmy so much as a puppy that when they had another litter we got another one. She's twelve now,"

Kathi told me that Emmy had been hefty for her breed, at seventy-three pounds, and she'd enjoyed pheasant hunting and obedience training.

In 2008, when Emmy was ten years old, the Streeters noticed the dog kept licking her right front leg. They took an x-ray in their clinic, spotted a mass, and immediately took the films to their neighbor, veterinarian Janet Lori, who was a resident at csu's veterinary cancer clinic at the time. Lori confirmed Emmy had osteosarcoma, and told the Streeters the Lab was an ideal fit for the new gene therapy trial, because she was strong and healthy, apart from her tumor, and her cancer had not metastasized. Lori explained that the dog would receive the gene therapy in conjunction with chemo, and then ten days later, her leg would be amputated.

Kathi admitted she was initially reluctant to enroll Emmy in the trial, because she was a cancer survivor herself, and she knew all too well what chemo was like. Kathi was fifty-four when, in 2004, she found a lump and learned it was a highly aggressive, metastatic breast tumor. She had a double mastectomy, followed by four months on an every-other-week chemo cocktail of doxorubicin and docetaxel. It was so hard on her body, she didn't believe she would make it out alive.

"I told Ron, 'They're just going to poison me to death,'" she said.

I understood her pessimism. I told her that I'd watched Beth lose her hair and waste away to ninety pounds. I'd listened to her insist she felt so sick she'd rather die than endure another round of chemo.

"I thought it would kind of be like it was for your sister. You get a diagnosis, you do what you can, and then a year later people are going to your funeral," said Kathi, who spoke about her cancer with an intimacy that had not faded, even though she had long passed the five-year cancer-free milestone that gave her the right to use that precious word that has eluded so many cancer patients: cured.

Her cure was a direct result of personalized medicine. As Kathi's four months of chemo were drawing to a close, the FDA approved Herceptin, a drug invented by the San Francisco–based company Genentech for patients whose breast tumors possessed the particular genetic mutation called HER2. Kathi tested positive for the mutation and immediately began receiving Herceptin intravenously every other week. After a year of treatment, Kathi was cancer-free. She believes she owes her life to Herceptin.

I told Kathi that while Beth was fighting her cancer in 2009, scientists proved that some stomach tumors also have the HER2 mutation. They found that Herceptin improved the survival of those patients by 37 percent over chemotherapy alone.[12] I had been elated when I found out Beth was being tested for the mutation, but my hope was short-lived — my sister's tumor was not HER2 positive.

"I felt really fortunate to have HER2. It gave me something I could do," Kathi said, tears welling in her eyes. "But as the years go on, I start feeling almost guilty I survived."

Herceptin was one of the first successes, along with Palladia and Sutent, in personalized medicine — drugs that obliterate tumors by targeting a specific genetic trait. Osteosarcoma was considered a prime candidate for personalized treatments, too, and dogs were helping to prove it. The company that brought Palladia to market, the Pfizer unit that was later named Zoetis, went on to develop a technique for predicting how dogs with osteosarcoma would respond to various therapy regimens based on the exact genetic makeup of their tumors. In a 2013 paper, they predicted a similar method could be adapted to benefit people with osteosarcoma.[13]

Gene therapy was another form of personalized medicine — one of many that was being perfected around that time. Just as CSU was completing its gene therapy trial, scientists at MD Anderson began researching a treatment in which they used dogs' own immune cells as weapons against their tumors. They simultaneously tested the therapy in children and adults with cancer. (For more on the MD Anderson research, see Chapter 5.)

But to perfect gene therapy, scientists needed more evidence that the basic technique worked on cancer —

evidence that would come from trials such as the one Kathi was offered as a last-ditch treatment for Emmy. Kathi quickly overcame her initial reluctance to volunteer Emmy for the trial: she knew she had to do it.

"I had gone through chemo and I survived," said Kathi, adding that she and Ron, who were both in their second marriages, had four children, six grandchildren, and two step-grandchildren between them. "If this were my child, it would be devastating. If we could learn something, we had to do it."

Emmy received doxorubicin during the chemo arm of her trial — the very same drug prescribed to Kathi. But Emmy didn't have any side effects, and the dog's attitude about her illness and treatment was far more positive than that of most people, including Kathi.

"I think part of it is because dogs don't worry about tomorrow," she said. "It's all about today. It was as if she were saying, 'Okay, stick a needle in me. Are you going to feed me? Do I get a bone then?'"

Emmy responded well to the gene therapy, chemo, and amputation, living an additional three years after the trial until she died of old age in 2011.

In December 2012, the team of vets who managed the gene therapy trial published their results. In their paper, they explained that they had tracked the activity of the inserted gene by measuring a protein associated with apoptosis. Far more of the tumor cells died in the dogs who received the experimental treatment than in the dogs who got chemotherapy alone.[14]

Eight of the fifty-six dogs who got the experimental

therapy were still alive after two hundred days, the researchers reported. There was no sign of cancer in any of them.

———

The dog trial was a small but important first step in what the participating scientists knew would be an arduous road to getting gene therapy approved to treat children with osteosarcoma. The challenges inherent in drug development were aptly illustrated by what happened to MTP-PE, the drug that was part of Emily Brown's life-saving regimen.

MTP-PE was shuttled through the initial stages of the development process by Eugenie Kleinerman, a pediatric oncologist at the MD Anderson Cancer Center, who managed several of the trials required to get regulatory approval for the drug around the world. Kleinerman had been interested in MTP-PE since the early 1980s, but back then she didn't have any good mouse models of osteosarcoma that she could use as evidence that it might work in people. So she kept a close eye on the work being done by the head of the University of Wisconsin's veterinary oncology program, Greg MacEwen, and the stellar results he was seeing in dogs with cancer.

"I found it invigorating that he had the same idea I did," Kleinerman told me when I phoned her to ask about MTP-PE. "Because you can move more rapidly into clinical testing in the veterinary world, it provided the validation that I needed for the pediatric community to pay attention."

After the positive results started piling up in children

with osteosarcoma, the Irvine, California–based company IDM Pharma took over the task of developing MTP-PE, and in 2009 won approval for the drug in Europe, where it went to market with the trade name Mepact. It was the first new treatment approved for osteosarcoma in twenty years,[15] and the achievement prompted Japan's Takeda Pharmaceutical Company to shell out $75 million to acquire IDM.

Because osteosarcoma affects fewer than two hundred thousand people per year, it's classified as an orphan disease. For decades, orphan diseases were all but ignored by the pharmaceutical industry. But that changed in the mid-2000s when drug companies started to recognize that life-saving treatments aimed at small patient populations could fetch high enough prices on the market to produce a significant return on investment. Perhaps more importantly, they also realized that such treatments could prove effective in treating other diseases down the road, expanding the market even more. This was particularly true for drugs used in oncology, where one scientific breakthrough — such as the ability to cut off the blood supply to tumors, which was so important to the success of Palladia and Sutent — can be applied to several types of cancers.

But Mepact faced a tough road to market in the United States. In 2007, the FDA requested that IDM perform a second clinical trial with nine hundred osteosarcoma patients — a trial that would take years to fill because of the rarity of the disease. IDM didn't have the resources to fund the trial, and as of 2014, Takeda hadn't committed to pursuing U.S. approval either.

Meanwhile, many of the children who had been lucky

enough to receive MTP-PE in the clinical trials were thriving. The pivotal study, which had begun in 1997, showed that when children with osteosarcoma received MTP-PE along with chemotherapy, the mortality rate eight years after diagnosis fell 30 percent. Fifteen years after diagnosis, that rate was still holding.[16] Even one of the earliest studies of MTP-PE, conducted in patients with osteosarcoma in the early 1990s, yielded remarkable survival rates — half the patients were still alive as of 2014, Kleinerman told me. Yet despite this proof of MTP-PE's power, the drug had not yet been approved in the United States because of the FDA's refusal to approve it without the second trial. That meant neither pediatricians nor veterinarians in the country where the drug was discovered and developed could get access to it — a failure that Kleinerman still found devastating.

"We've made a lot of progress in surgery, a lot of progress in the diagnostic imaging," Kleinerman said. "But we really are at a standstill in terms of [drug] treatment."

I asked Withrow what motivated him to continue working on behalf of pets and children with cancer when there were so many obstacles, so many disappointments. He told me that at the beginning of his career at CSU, he volunteered every summer at the Sky High Hope Camp, a week-long camp in Bellvue, Colorado, for kids with cancer and their siblings. Every year he went, he said, he was inspired by the children he met there, whom he knew could benefit from his work in dogs.

One of those children was Emily Brown. In 1999, Withrow arrived at the camp and recognized Emily, who was then thirteen and had finished her cancer treatments.

Withrow introduced himself, and told her he had contributed to her treatment. Emily thought he was joking.

"I said, 'I have no idea who you are. You're a vet. I'm a human. Obviously you've never been involved in my care,'" Emily recalled.

Withrow explained to her that MTP-PE had originally been tested in pet dogs, and her oncologists at Denver Children's had consulted with him about the drug. Emily still didn't believe him — her oncologist, Gore, had mentioned animal studies but not in enough detail for her to fully understand what had happened. So Withrow invited her to visit CSU's animal cancer center to see exactly how his patients had helped her. She took him up on the offer.

"The comparison between animal and human [biology] was never even a blip on my mental radar," said Emily, who spent a day at CSU attending rounds with the veterinarians and meeting the dogs who were there for treatment.

She was so enchanted by the experience that she went back several years later for a college internship. She wrote stories for the center's newsletter about canine cancer survivors and their families.

"It's more than just the biology that translates so well. It's the actual care they're giving the animals," she said. "It was just like being in a children's hospital, with all the caretakers — the nurses, the doctors, the residents. That's what I loved. The absolute correlation between the two was astounding."

Whenever Withrow reflected on all the years he'd spent looking for cures for osteosarcoma, he often harkened back to his training in the 1970s, when the prognosis for children with the disease was so bleak oncologists were still quoting a line uttered in 1955 by a physician named Stanford Cade.[17]

"Gentlemen, if we operate they die. If we don't operate they die," Cade said during a conference for oncologists specializing in osteosarcoma. "This meeting should be concluded with prayer."

Partnering with dogs, Withrow predicted, would prove more effective than pleading for divine intervention in osteosarcoma.

"Kids are direct beneficiaries of what we learn in animals," Withrow said. "I can see them running around at camp, enjoying life, alive. That's why I'm doing this."

Chapter 5
A Golden Opportunity
to Cure Lymphoma

During my trip to Colorado State, I stopped by the home of Danielle Balogh, who had enrolled her golden retriever, Maya, in a study at CSU in 2012, after the dog was diagnosed with lymphoma. Maya, a playful six-year-old with white highlights in the fur on her face, was assigned to receive one of three novel chemotherapy agents that had been developed by the National Cancer Institute. Maya spent nearly a week at CSU, getting infusions of the drug, and having her blood tested and tumors tracked to determine her response. The CSU vets quickly discovered that the experimental drug wasn't shrinking the dog's tumors, so they took Maya off it and put her on an older chemotherapy regimen instead. She was in remission when I met her.

"We weren't disappointed at all," Balogh said, as the dog dashed around her small apartment, playing with an Angry Birds squeaky toy. "We hadn't set her back any further by doing the study. And hopefully she's going to help someone, or some dog, somehow."

Lymphoma is a type of blood cancer that affects lymphocytes, the white blood cells that are part of the immune system's guard against infections. Several breeds are prone to it, including cocker spaniels, Siberian huskies, Shih Tzus, and bassett hounds,[1] but no breed has been harder hit by lymphoma than the golden retriever. About one out of every eight goldens will develop lymphoma at some point in his or her lifetime.[2]

The most common type of lymphoma in dogs is similar to non–Hodgkin's lymphoma (NHL), a disease that newly affects seventy thousand Americans each year.[3] NHL claims about twenty thousand lives every year, making it the sixth deadliest cancer. It's also one of the few forms of the disease that's becoming more prevalent over time.[4]

The rising rate of NHL is one of the many mysteries surrounding this cancer. Age seems to be the only obvious risk factor for it — most lymphoma cases occur in people over sixty. Some studies suggest that exposure to insecticides may be the cause, but that evidence hasn't been widely validated. And NHL is more prevalent in men than women, especially in Caucasian men who live in developed countries. No one knows why.[5]

When dogs get this type of lymphoma, they are typically prescribed the same chemo treatments that people get, and many are fated to the same sad consequence: resistance, progression, death.

Balogh and her husband, Kyle, had purchased Maya as a puppy when they were both attending college in Denver. Five years later, they were just starting life as a married couple — still paying off student loans and building a house — when Kyle felt a lump on Maya's neck. The dog was like a child to the newlyweds, so they were willing to do everything to save her life, but they were worried about how they would pay for the treatments.

The trial that Maya was invited to join was designed to determine if any of three experimental chemo agents called indenoisoquinolines would be effective in fighting lymphoma, and if so, what dosage would work best. Sue Lana, the CSU veterinarian who was managing the trial there, told me that the information gathered from the dogs was helping oncologists move more quickly through human trials, which were happening simultaneously.

CSU offered the Baloghs a $1,000 credit toward Maya's treatments as part of the study, guaranteeing that if the dog didn't do well on whichever of the three experimental drugs she was randomly assigned to receive, they could use the money to try something else. It was a huge relief for the young couple.

"The funds gave us a jump-start to do the chemo," Balogh said.

When Balogh found out that the results of Lana's research would be used to help humans with the disease, she knew she had made the right decision to enroll Maya in the trial. One of Balogh's closest friends had been diagnosed with Hodgkin's lymphoma around the time of Maya's diagnosis. Both went through chemo at the same time, and both were doing well, Balogh told me. With perfect timing, Maya trotted up to me and put her head in my lap.

"I'm sorry you're going through this cancer," I said to the dog.

Balogh echoed my sympathy and admitted it was often hard for her to tell how Maya was feeling. Then she repeated a sentiment I had heard many times before from dog owners participating in comparative oncology studies. She told me she believed her dog's ordeal was serving a higher purpose.

"You're so cool, Maya," she said, picking up one of the dog's tennis balls and rolling it across the floor for a game of fetch. "You're helping people."

The idea that golden retrievers can contribute something special to the betterment of human health got a major push in the summer of 2012 from the Morris Animal Foundation, a Denver-based non-profit that supports research to improve veterinary medicine. That's when Morris launched the Golden Retriever Lifetime Study, a project designed to track three thousand golden retrievers for more than ten years, recording everything about the dogs' lives: their diets, the environment in which they live, how much they exercise, the diseases they develop, and whether they pass a susceptibility to those illnesses along to their puppies — who, ideally, are also enrolled in the study as they arrive.

When I met Rod Page at csu, he was pulling double duty, taking over the directorship of the university's veterinary cancer center while at the same time managing the Morris Foundation's study. He told me that one of the major goals of the research, which was funded by $25 million in donations, was to determine why more than half of all goldens die from lymphoma and other cancers. He believed that insight would be directly applicable to human oncology research.

"There will be plenty of opportunity for translational studies related to common exposures — genetics, diet, and other influences," he said. "We can study these issues in dogs sometimes better than we can in people."

The pet owners who enrolled in the study agreed to bring their dogs to their local vets every year for physical exams, during which tissue samples — blood, urine, fur, toenail clippings, and more — would be collected and mailed to the investigators. The owners also filled out an extensive online questionnaire, and agreed that when their pets died they would consider a necropsy (the veterinary equivalent of an autopsy), so the researchers could further investigate the factors that contributed to each dog's demise.

The designers of the Golden Retriever Lifetime Study modeled their research after similar long-term studies done in humans, most notably the Framingham Heart Study. The Framingham project, named after the Massachusetts town where it started in 1948, kicked off with 5,209 volunteers between the ages of thirty and sixty-two, who all agreed to share their medical records with the project throughout their lives. The study — which is jointly managed by the National Heart, Lung, and Blood Institute and Boston University — is ongoing, and has since enrolled more than five thousand children and grandchildren of the original volunteers.[6]

Data from Framingham has completely reshaped how physicians manage and prevent cardiovascular disease by better defining how such risk factors as high cholesterol, diabetes, age, and gender contribute to heart health.

"When we talk about our study," Page said of the golden retriever research, "we call it the Framingham Study for dogs."

———

The role of companion dogs in helping improve the outlook for lymphoma patients dates back to the 1960s, when two oncologists at the Fred Hutchinson Cancer Center in Seattle, Rainer Storb and E. Donnall Thomas, were perfecting bone marrow transplants for treating blood-borne cancers in humans. Their plan was to use chemotherapy to kill off the cancer cells, then take marrow donated by healthy people and inject it into patients' veins. Once the stem cells in the healthy marrow found their way to the patients' bones, they would churn out normal blood cells in perpetuity.

The idea of treating cancer patients with marrow from healthy donors had been around for a decade or so at that point, and it had been widely tested in rodents, Storb told me. But when the technique was tried in people, it didn't work. The problem, he said, was that oncologists didn't know how to prevent patients' immune systems from rejecting the donated marrow. Thomas and Storb believed dogs could help them figure it out.

Why dogs? The two physicians were intrigued by the phenotypic diversity of dogs, Storb said, referring to the vast differences that exist within the canine species, not just in how their genes are expressed to create a wide variety of traits, but also in how those genes interact with the environment.

"Think of a tiny Chihuahua all the way up to a Great Dane. Dogs have a lot of phenotypic diversity, just like humans," he said.

So in 1966, Storb drew up a letter and mailed it to veterinarians all over the West Coast. It explained that they wanted to try to cure dogs of NHL using experimental bone-marrow transplantation regimens. Much to his surprise, more than 1,500 dog owners volunteered for the research.

Over the next few years, Storb and Thomas figured out how to pre-treat the dogs with radiation to suppress their immune systems and prevent rejection of the donated marrow. Then they devised chemotherapy regimens that would boost the probability of the transplants succeeding. Of the initial dogs they treated, Storb said, about 30 percent were cured. A control group of eight dogs who received only chemotherapy didn't do nearly as well; all of them relapsed and died within nine months.

One of the most important advances from Storb and Thomas's dog trials was that they helped define the concept of histocompatibility typing — a process by which substances on the surface of cells called antigens are matched between donor and recipient to further decrease the chance of rejection. In the early days of bone marrow transplantation, oncologists believed that only siblings or other family members could be histocompatible. It was Storb and his colleagues who proved, first in dogs and then in people, that unrelated donors could also be compatible. They reported their finding in the late 1970s,[7] and shortly thereafter, they achieved their first successful human bone marrow transplant from a non-relative to a patient with leukemia.

The effort to refine bone marrow transplantation involved a small but dedicated team of oncologists and veterinarians, who set up shop in an abandoned World War II military bunker outside of Seattle, Storb said. Veterinarians who were members of the United States Army Reserve often showed up on weekends and volunteered to help with the dogs. The human patients, who were also treated at that site, were usually greeted by a cacophony of barking as they pulled into the parking lot, but they didn't find that strange at all.

"They were aware of the fact that the treatments they received were pioneered in dogs, so they were perfectly accepting of it," Storb said.

Today there are more than ten million potential bone marrow donors in the United States registered with the National Marrow Donor Program.[8] The organization facilitates nearly 500 transplants per month on average for patients suffering from one of a number of diseases, including all the major forms of lymphoma and leukemia. Thomas received the Nobel Prize for his pioneering work on organ and cell transplantation in 1990, and after his death in 2012, Storb carried on the work in bone marrow transplants, launching new trials in dogs and people designed to improve the technique even further.

———

I wanted to learn more about how dogs with lymphoma were helping people, so a few months after I visited CSU, I traveled to the school that first introduced me to comparative oncology: Texas A&M University in College Station. It was A&M veterinary surgeon Theresa Fossum who had sat in my office in New York and told me that pets get many of the same cancers humans do. Fossum had invited me to the state-of-the-art veterinary research center that opened at A&M in 2007. So that's where I started my visit.

The research center, called the Texas A&M Institute for Preclinical Studies (TIPS), was the newest addition to the university's ninety-year-old veterinary school, which I was surprised to learn is the only one in Texas. The school, which treats ninety thousand animals per year, offers a number of services in one location.[9] In addition to TIPS, the teaching facilities, and full-service hospitals for large and small animals, Texas A&M is home to the Stevenson Companion Animal Life-Care Center, which houses pets whose owners pre-decease them or who have to leave them behind when they enter nursing homes. When I got there, the school had just raised $120 million to build a new educational wing and to expand the small-animal hospital.[10]

TIPS was designed as a one-stop shop for developers of new drugs and medical devices. The 112,000-square-foot facility provides services for researchers who want to study pets with naturally occurring diseases such as cancer. It includes a business incubator for life sciences start-ups, some of which were founded based on science developed at the university. And TIPS also houses — and sometimes develops — the animal models traditionally used in scientific research, such as rodents with human diseases.

Fossum, TIPS's director at the time, told me that putting all the steps of product development in one place was a good way to ensure that companion animals would get access to cutting-edge treatments, even if those treatments were being developed for people.

"I have always had an interest in trying to take the experimental work that we do and make sure that animals with naturally occurring diseases are used where it's appropriate," she said. "Whenever possible, I want to translate all the wonderful things coming through here that are meant for people into products that can help dogs or cats."

Texas A&M also wanted to offer the most advanced capabilities it could for medical imaging, so the university hired Mark Lenox, who had played a key role in the development of Positron Emission Tomography (PET) imaging technology. PET, which didn't really take off until it was combined with computed tomography (CT) scanning around 2000, offers oncologists and scientists the ability to see inside the body in ways not possible before, using nuclear imaging to bring to light the most intricate structures — from muscle to brain tissue — and to improve the ability to precisely measure tumor shrinkage and other effects of cancer therapies.

Lenox, an engineer who spent much of his career at German medical-devices giant Siemens, was retired when he heard about TIPS. He and his wife, both Texas A&M graduates, decided if there was any job worth coming out of retirement for, it would be this one, he told me while we walked through an enormous lecture hall toward the imaging suite that housed one iteration of the PET machine he helped develop. His job at Texas A&M was to take that basic technology and adapt it to a range of animal studies, he explained, as he pulled up PET scans of a dog named Rowdy on a large computer outside the imaging suite.

"When a company comes here with a question or a problem, it's all about a measurement they want to make," Lenox said. It's something they want to identify, like whether a drug is going where it's supposed to go and not anywhere else."

Oftentimes, he explained, those techniques had not yet been invented, so Lenox would write special software for the PET scanner to provide the quality of image a researcher was requesting.

Rowdy, a Great Pyrenees, was part of a trial of a new device that delivered radiation straight to bone tumors. The technique, called brachytherapy, wasn't new — implantable radioactive seeds have long been used to shrink tumors, particularly in prostate cancer — but it hadn't really caught on as a treatment for osteosarcoma. Then Houston engineer Stan Stearns approached Texas A&M with a tiny drill he'd invented that could make miniscule holes in bone and then deposit a radioactive particle straight to the tumor. Texas A&M agreed to be the primary testing site for the device.

Lenox pulled up Rowdy's images on twin computer screens and clicked through them until he hit upon a bright white mass, the tumor, surrounded by even brighter pinpricks — the tiny holes used to inject the radiation. On the PET scan, the veterinarians leading the trials could see the radioactive particle, yttrium-90, as it made its way to the tumor, Lenox explained.

"The difficulty in brachytherapy is getting the right amount in the right place. We can see where the yttrium-90 is while it's actually doing its work on the tumor," he said.

Stearns's invention was the result of a personal mission. The founder and president of a Houston-based maker of industrial instruments, Stearns had lost his dog, Gabriel, in 2008, after a year-long quest to find a cure for the dog's osteosarcoma. Stearns had brought Gabriel — a sweet-tempered, smaller-than-average Saint Bernard — to both CSU and UC Davis for treatment. It was during that time that he dreamed up the radiation drill, later using his engineering skills to make it a reality. He believed the drill could ultimately help humans with osteosarcoma. Stearns launched his own foundation, the Gabriel Institute, to raise money to develop the drill and contribute to other research projects to help dogs and people with cancer.

"I wanted to do something more than just [fund-raising] walks," Stearns told me when I met him at his office near Houston. "Everyone is touched by cancer in some way. In my case, my passion was turned on by a dog."

Rowdy didn't survive — his cancer spread to his lungs — and when I met Stearns, he was still working with Texas A&M to improve upon the brachytherapy device.

To the veterinary school's dean, Eleanor Green, persisting despite such struggles was vital to the school's mission. Halfway through my Texas trip, I sat down with her to talk about Texas A&M's responsibilities as the only veterinary school in the state.

"Texas is a state of 25 million people. It's number one in the nation in [population of] beef cattle and horses," said Green, a native Floridian who spent most of her career as an equine medicine specialist before moving into academia. "That gives us a tremendous opportunity and obligation to serve societal needs, not only in this state but in the nation."

Green told me she was attracted to A&M for the way its students, or "Aggies" upheld school traditions. One of those is the school's official mascot, Reveille, a position currently served by a rough collie. A portrait of Reveille — named for a stray adopted by a group of student cadets in 1931 — hangs in the vet school. Aggies are notoriously loyal to their traditions, Green explained, and they follow an honor code that imbues them with a sense of responsibility to their chosen professions.

Green added that Texas A&M is an enthusiastic participant in One Health, an international program designed to foster collaborations among medical professionals that could benefit both animal and human health. The school is in a unique position to work with physicians who develop therapies for people, Green said, because of its proximity to Texas Medical Center — a sprawling Houston campus encompassing twenty-one hospitals, including MD Anderson Cancer Center, the Texas Heart Institute, and Texas Children's Hospital.

"We're ninety miles from the largest medical center in the world," Green said. "Once we all recognize what everyone brings to the table and the synergies that occur, you can't stop us."

In 2008, Texas A&M veterinarian Heather Wilson-Robles went to MD Anderson to lead a seminar on comparative oncology. The soft-spoken veterinarian, who had only begun practicing five years earlier, was so intimidated by the intellectual firepower in that room she thought she might puke.

"I sat down in a room with all these MDs and they're all staring at me," she told me. "There I was, this little veterinarian. What did I know?"

Wilson-Robles soon discovered, much to her surprise, that many of the oncologists at MD Anderson knew much less than she did about dogs and cancer — in fact, they knew nothing.

"They were like, 'Dogs get cancer? No way!'" Wilson-Robles said. "We started talking more about the similarities between dogs and people with cancer, and they began to realize this was an excellent model."

A week later, Wilson-Robles's phone rang. It was Laurence Cooper, associate director of immunology at MD Anderson. He told her he'd been thinking of taking immune cells from patients with lymphoma and using them as weapons against their disease. This would be the ultimate in personalized medicine — a therapy that was individualized to each patient, designed to mobilize that patient's own immune system to defeat his or her cancer. Cooper wanted first to try the idea on dogs with lymphoma to find out if it could work. What's more, he wanted to treat the dogs using the same meticulous standards practiced in human clinical trials at MD Anderson, where more than 115,000 people from around the world came every year to be treated with the latest cancer therapies available.

Cooper's idea centered on T cells, white blood cells that play a key role in the immune system's ability to hunt down pathogens in the body and kill them. He told Wilson-Robles that his plan was to remove T cells from the blood of dogs with lymphoma, grow those cells in the lab, then infuse them back into the dogs along with a standard chemotherapy treatment. He believed that therapy would be enough to prolong their survival. Ultimately, his goal was to genetically engineer the T cells to give them even more cancer-killing power.

I asked Wilson-Robles to explain how such a therapy might work, and she told me to think of the immune system as an army, with a hierarchy of cells that have specific roles in fighting disease. Some immune cells are like generals, she said, because they tell all the other white blood cells what to do. Others, including cytotoxic T cells, also known as CD8 lymphocytes, are the foot soldiers that go out and kill diseased cells such as B cells, which have been implicated in the most common type of non-Hodgkin's lymphoma.

"What happens in cancer is the ratio goes out of whack, so there are too many generals and not enough soldiers," Wilson-Robles explained. By taking the T cells out, growing them and putting them back into the body, "we have a lot more soldiers and very few generals."

Wilson-Robles was enthusiastic about Cooper's idea and started a trial for dogs with lymphoma, working closely with MD Anderson biologist Colleen O'Connor, who was responsible for treating the dogs and cultivating their

T cells. I visited O'Connor at her lab, which was filled with photos of the dogs in the trial. They included a champion Rottweiler and a seeing-eye dog who came all the way from the Netherlands with his owner to receive the treatment. She considered all of them to be like her children, she said.

Having lost a dog to cancer herself, O'Connor had great sympathy for the owners of her canine patients. O'Connor told me that she and her family in Kentucky often drove their elderly bichon three hours each way to Ohio State University during the dog's battle with cancer, so she could be treated by the region's top cancer specialists.

"I understand these people, because I've lived through it," O'Connor said.

T cell therapies had been tried in human patients before, but when techniques that were developed in mice were translated to people, they often didn't work. They were far too toxic — igniting what's known as a cytokine storm, which is a potentially fatal immune reaction — and they rarely did much to beat back the cancer. The MD Anderson team developed a protocol that involved pre-treating the cancer with chemotherapy and fine-tuning the concentration of T cells used, so they would do their work without sparking a dangerous immune response.

O'Connor marveled at the dedication of the dog owners to the idea of treating their pets' disease with a new and unproven technique. All participants in the trial had to have blood samples collected from their dogs once a week and sent to her, so she could track the activity of the transplanted T cells.

"The owners would pay to go to their own vets, have the

samples taken and then send them to me," O'Connor said. "Do you know how great that is? It shows how much they loved their dogs."

One of O'Connor's volunteers was Shelley Robson, who worked as a fundraiser in MD Anderson's development office. When Robson's thirteen-year-old boxer mix, Dutch, was diagnosed with B-cell lymphoma, she immediately called O'Connor's lab and asked if she could put her dog in the trial.

Dutch was a sweet-tempered, fifty-five-pound ball of muscle, who enjoyed accompanying Robson and her husband to a local bar called the Gingerman, where the dog was known for his ability to lap up an entire can of Guinness in one sitting. Any time he heard a siren near the dog park, he would draw laughs by howling along, and he once won a Halloween costume contest dressed as Muhammad Ali, with baby-sized boxing gloves around his neck and a t-shirt picturing a butterfly and a bee.

By the time Dutch's cancer was discovered, it had already spread to his spleen. Robson's vet told her he had just six weeks to live, so she decided to give the T cells a try, not only to help Dutch but also to advance the research, which she knew from her five years of working at MD Anderson would somehow end up helping people with cancer. Whenever she ran into O'Connor at work, Robson told me, the scientist would insist that they go back to her lab to check how Dutch's T cells were doing.

"She was like a proud mama," Robson said. "We'd look at the cells under a microscope. She'd ask me if Dutch was eating and getting his medicine on time."

Dutch succumbed to his cancer in March 2012. Robson figured the trial gave the dog an additional seven months of life.

"We felt like we were able to contribute to the science without causing him to suffer," she said. "Up until the end he was playing, just like a puppy. The seven months we got were really good ones."

When MD Anderson and Texas A&M published the results of the trial in February 2012, they revealed that the dogs who got the T cell treatment had a median overall survival rate of 392 days — more than twice that of historical controls, which were dogs who in the past had been treated with chemo alone.[11]

MD Anderson went on to launch a trial of T cells in people, which involved not just cultivating the cells after they were removed, but also tweaking them to improve their cancer-hunting abilities. The technique uses a method of genetic engineering called Sleeping Beauty, in which a therapeutic gene is introduced into the DNA of a patient's T cells. Once in place, the gene produces a protein, called a chimeric antigen receptor (CAR), that helps T cells spot the patient's cancer cells and destroy them. (The method was dubbed Sleeping Beauty because it originally involved a dormant gene found in fish that scientists brought back to life and engineered to perform a therapeutic job.[12])

To better explain how Sleeping Beauty works, O'Connor took out a piece of paper and began to draw. Instead of using generals and soldiers as an analogy, O'Connor compared a cancer cell to a woman wearing a ball gown at a baseball game. If the T cell recognizes the woman as a healthy cell, it won't kill her, even though the ball gown makes her look a little out of place. The CAR protein allows the T cell to recognize that the ball gown is actually a tumor fingerprint — a signal that the cell needs to be eliminated.

With the help of the CAR, O'Connor said, the engineered T cell says, "'Whoa, that's a *blue* ball gown. That's foreign, and we're not going to allow that.'"

MD Anderson's scientists envisioned expanding the role of T cells in the personalization of cancer therapy, and they continued to rely on dogs to provide supporting evidence for their ideas. In a subsequent trial, O'Connor gave stem cell transplants to dogs with B-cell lymphoma, followed by injections of their own T cells. The goal was to see if the cells might boost the success rate of stem cell transplantation, which is still commonly used to treat lymphoma in people, even though half of patients eventually relapse. It worked, O'Connor said, providing an early but promising sign that the key to curing cancer may lie in each patient's innate power to fight off disease.

"Our ultimate achievement would be to cure cancer with these cells. That's what we're really trying to do," O'Connor said. "And we're trying to do it without the use of chemo and radiation."

———

For all the medical advances being made in the fight against lymphoma, there is a whole set of questions yet to be answered. What causes this cancer? Why is its incidence increasing over time? What secrets are buried in the

genes of patients and their family members that may lead
to more personalized treatments in the future? Those questions, and the eventual answers, might prove applicable to
all cancers.

In the summer of 2013, shortly after I returned from
Texas A&M, I discovered a research project similar to the
Golden Retriever Lifetime Study — but this time on the
human side. It was the American Cancer Society's Cancer
Prevention Study, a multi-year effort to track 300,000
healthy Americans throughout their lifetimes, with the
ultimate goal of gaining new insights into what causes cancer and what might prevent it.

I volunteered for the study by logging on to its website and filling out a fifteen-part questionnaire that covered everything from what vitamins I was taking, to how
much sun I had been exposed to throughout my life, to
how much physical activity I was getting during the typical
work day.

When I got to the "family history" section, I stopped,
confused by my choices. The questionnaire asked if I have
any siblings. Under "sister" I marked "1." Beth is gone, but
she's still a part of my history, I figured. Then I was asked
to reveal if any parents or siblings had been diagnosed with
cancer. I checked off "yes," then typed in "gastric cancer."

The questionnaire didn't ask if any of my siblings had
survived cancer, nor could I find any checkbox for the
number of siblings who had died. I found this strange, so I
went back through the other sections of the survey, just in
case I'd missed it — the opportunity to reveal the unspeakable toll this disease took on my family. It wasn't there.

A week or so later I was summoned to the Cancer Society's Hope Lodge in New York, where I gave up seven teaspoons of blood and had my blood pressure, heart rate, and waist circumference measured. I signed a consent form that explained my blood sample would be frozen and used "for future analyses of genetic and biologic markers of disease," which might then be used to create new medicines or diagnostic tests. I was promised a regular newsletter, which would update me on any published results from the study. And I vowed I would periodically fill out a new questionnaire, so the researchers could be kept up-to-date on any change in the state of my health.

As I left Hope Lodge, I couldn't help but think that I had, in my own small way, made a contribution to cancer research. After all, if those three thousand golden retrievers could give blood samples once a year for the benefit of finding a cure, surely I could do it this one time. If all those dog owners could take an hour out of their day every once in a while to report how their four-legged friends were faring, I could also take the time to update the American Cancer Society's researchers about my health.

I have to believe that with the participation of all of us — oncologists, veterinarians, men, women, children, dogs — science will ultimately find better ways to prevent cancer, and will discover more Sleeping Beauties to cure the next generation of patients.

Chapter 6
Cali's Total Mastectomy

Mildred Edmond was browsing through photos of adoptable pets on the website of an animal shelter near her home in suburban Philadelphia just after Thanksgiving in 2009 when she first saw Cali. Edmond was immediately taken in by the shy gaze of the bichon-poodle mix with the bright white, curly coat. It wasn't as if Edmond needed another dog — she and her husband, Ron, already had their hands full with their cockapoo, P.J., and poodle mix, Farah. But Edmond couldn't shake the hunch that she and Cali were meant to be together. So she dragged her husband to the shelter to meet the dog.

When the Edmonds arrived at the SPCA they learned about Cali's troubled past. The dog, who was about six, had been rescued from a puppy mill in Lancaster, Pennsylvania, where she had spent her life in a cage, producing litter after litter. Her feet were permanently webbed from her years pacing the cage's wire floor, and anxiety had driven her to chew her paws raw, leaving them covered in painful cysts. She had lost all but four of her teeth.

Cali also had tumors in all but one of her mammary glands. Her diagnosis was carcinoma in situ, which meant her cancer had not spread beyond her mammary glands and was likely curable with surgery. But she would need to be closely monitored for the rest of her life. Just as women who are diagnosed with breast carcinoma in situ face a two- to four-times increased risk of developing invasive breast cancer down the road,[1] dogs with the same tumor type in their mammary glands are also in danger of eventually facing a much deadlier cancer.

Edmond learned that Cali had been accepted into a comparative trial at the University of Pennsylvania in Philadelphia, where veterinarians were studying canine mammary tumors, hoping to gain new insights into human breast cancer. Penn's veterinary clinic would treat the dog at no charge to whomever agreed to give her a home.

Edmond — who herself had beaten breast cancer five years earlier — knew she had to help this dog. She and her husband adopted Cali, and just before Christmas they drove from their home in Warminster, Pennsylvania, to the Ryan Veterinary Hospital on Penn's campus to embark on Cali's cancer treatment.

On my way to Penn to learn about the mammary tumor study, I stopped at Edmond's home, which faced a traffic-filled street in a bustling working-class neighborhood dotted with Dairy Queens and Wawa convenience stores. When Edmond opened the door to let me in, P.J. and Farah came running, wagging their tails and taking turns jumping up to greet me.

Edmond, a petite woman, scolded her dogs playfully, but with just enough authority to get them to obey. "Down! Be nice! Get in your house!"

Her dogs understood that "house" meant their crates, which were lined up neatly in the living room, each one furnished with cushions and blankets and their doors always left open. Whenever she needed to herd the dogs away from visitors she'd say, "Get in your house!" and they'd go in and poke their heads out the front, waiting eagerly for a treat or an invitation to join the guests on the couch.

Edmond picked up Cali, who was cowering at her feet.

"She's still shy," Edmond said. "When we first brought her home, she pulled back when we went to pick her up. That's because of the way she was brought up."

The veterinarians at Penn had removed all of Cali's mammary glands, and by the time I met her, the scars had faded and were covered with silky fur. There was no sign of cancer anywhere in her body, Edmond said.

I sat down on Edmond's couch, peering into Cali's enormous eyes and stroking her curly coat, and we talked about the bond that forms between dog and owner when both have survived the same disease.

"I've been clean eight years now," Edmond said, as she pulled down the front of her tank top to show me the scar across her right breast, a constant reminder of the lumpectomy, radiation, and chemotherapy that cured her cancer. Edmond said she feared that her two granddaughters might face a high risk for breast cancer, and she was grateful to Cali, she said, for contributing to research that might lead to better methods of detection and treatment.

"I didn't know that dogs get almost the same cancer as us," Edmond said. "Poor little Cali. She had a total mastectomy."

Mammary tumors are the most prevalent form of cancer in female dogs, accounting for half of all cancer diagnoses.[2] The incidence of mammary cancer is higher in dogs than in any other domesticated animal, and three times higher than it is in humans, where despite advances in chemotherapy and surgery, it remains second only to lung cancer as the biggest cancer killer of women.[3]

Mammary cancer bears remarkable similarities to breast cancer. For example, mammary tumors in dogs are often driven by hormones like estrogen, as some breast cancers are. And the BRCA1 and BRCA2 genetic mutations that predispose women to breast cancer have also been found in English springer spaniels with mammary tumors.[4]

Penn's mammary tumor research program was started in 2009 by Karin Sorenmo, an oncologist at the university's veterinary school, who came up with the idea when she was on a sabbatical in her home country of Norway. She told me that spaying and neutering, except for medical reasons, is illegal in Norway, where pet overpopulation has never been a problem. That makes female dogs there especially prone to mammary tumors — a danger they share with women who develop breast cancer.

"The risk of developing breast cancer in women is dependent on the dose of hormones they get over a lifetime. Same in dogs," Sorenmo said.

Research has shown that women who start menstruating before age twelve or who go through menopause after age fifty five have a higher risk of breast cancer, likely because of their longer-than-average exposure to estrogen and progesterone. Women who use hormones for birth control or to relieve hot flashes and other menopause symptoms also face a higher risk.[5] Similarly, female dogs who are not spayed before they first go into heat have a higher lifetime exposure to estrogen and progesterone than spayed dogs do, which greatly increases their risk of mammary cancer: The incidence of mammary tumors in dogs who experience just one heat is as high as 26 percent, whereas the risk in dogs who are spayed before they go into heat is a low 0.5 percent.[6]

While in Norway, Sorenmo saw mammary cancer in all its stages in the dogs she was treating, from benign nodules that could be easily removed to aggressively metastatic masses that had spread far beyond the mammary glands. Often these quite different tumors appeared in the same dog, a phenomenon Sorenmo recognized as a potential boon to breast cancer research.

"The dog provides us a snapshot of the entire continuum, from benign to malignant," Sorenmo said. "If you can study all the various steps, you can ask what are the most important molecular events that happen in dogs that develop malignant tumors."

Dogs are also ideal research partners because they usually have ten mammary glands, Sorenmo explained. Most dogs diagnosed with mammary cancer have tumors in some but not all of those glands, and a little less than half those tumors are malignant by the time their owners bring the dog to the vet to be diagnosed.[7] Veterinarians routinely remove the healthy glands along with the diseased ones to protect the animal from any recurrence of cancer. That gives them the rare opportunity to compare diseased and healthy mammary tissue from the same patient.

"We know that women who have benign breast lesions have an increased risk for developing breast cancer later, in the same breast, as well as in the other breast. That tells us that something has changed overall in the breast tissue that's a predictor for later breast cancer," Sorenmo said. "But it's difficult to study this progression in women because we have only two breasts."

Indeed, it's often not feasible to expect a woman undergoing a biopsy or a lumpectomy for an early-stage cancer to agree to volunteer to have healthy breast tissue removed for the benefit of a study. While many women who have had tumors in one breast or who face a high genetic risk of breast cancer sometimes have preventative mastectomies of healthy breasts, it's unlikely those tissues would show the full progression from benign to malignant. It is possible to compare breast samples taken from different women — and plenty of breast cancer studies are designed that way — but that's not ideal, Sorenmo said.

"If you were to take breast tissue from me and you and compare it, there would be a lot of differences because we are different individuals," Sorenmo said. "The advantage in the dog is that you can actually study this in the same individual."

When Sorenmo returned to Penn, she approached local shelters and rescue groups, asking them to keep an eye open for dogs with mammary tumors who had been abandoned. Then one day a geneticist from nearby Princeton

University named Olga Troyanskaya came to Sorenmo's clinic with her thirteen-year-old German shepherd, Jessy, who was suffering from cancer that had spread to her liver. Troyanskaya's regular vet had told her Jessy had only two weeks to live; with the help of a chemo regimen prescribed by Sorenmo, the dog gained six months of quality life.

As Sorenmo treated Jessy, she talked with Troyanskaya about her plan to study tumor samples from dogs with mammary cancer. Troyanskaya, who had researched human breast cancer at Princeton, volunteered to analyze the dog tissues for molecular differences between benign and the malignant tumors and then to look for similarities in tissue samples taken from women with breast cancer.

"By itself, molecular analysis is not so useful. You need clinical data to see what happened with each dog," Sorenmo said. "We planned to merge our information, so we could see which molecular changes predicted which dogs would develop malignancies later. Then we would compare that with human breast cancer data."

It didn't take long for word to spread around Philadelphia that Sorenmo was looking to rescue and treat dogs with mammary tumors. Soon patients started arriving, and by the time I visited her, three years after the start of her research, she had treated nearly seventy abandoned dogs. All of them had since found homes.

—

Penn's veterinary school was both foreign and familiar to me. I was an undergraduate there, and I spent half of my college years on campus living in dorms in a high-rise complex that was a short walk from the veterinary school. But I had never ventured into the animal clinic, which was part of a sprawling medical complex that includes two of the world's leaders in oncology research — Children's Hospital of Philadelphia and Abramson Cancer Center. Now, deeply entrenched in my search for hope in dogs, I was eager to see how my alma mater was contributing to comparative oncology.

Penn's veterinary school handles more than thirty-one thousand appointments for dogs and cats per year, a third of which come through its 24/7 emergency room.[8] This urban clinic is too compact to accommodate cows and horses, though, so Penn maintains a second veterinary campus on seven hundred acres in Kennett Square, Pennsylvania, a rural community thirty-six miles west of the main campus. The veterinarians and students who work there manage four thousand patient visits per year on site, in addition to treating thirty-one thousand animals on local farms.[9]

Penn's small-animal clinic offers a range of services that are not widely available elsewhere, including kidney transplants and dialysis, and it houses a specialty clinic for exotic animals. When I was there, students concentrating on exotics were treating a black-eyed white ferret for gall bladder disease and hepatitis, and an iguana who was recovering from surgery to remove her ovaries, which had been blocked by dozens of egg follicles.

Penn's veterinarians recruit dogs, cats, and sometimes even iguanas for trials that fall into four research priorities: infectious disease, neurology, regenerative medicine, and cancer. In addition to the mammary tumor program, the clinic was running ongoing trials in end-stage cancer pain and cancer cachexia — severe weight loss that's common in people and cats with cancer — when I was there.

Dorothy "Dottie" Brown, Penn's director of veterinary clinical investigations, told me the school always found plenty of volunteers for comparative trials, but that all pet owners are put through a careful screening process to ensure they can handle the requirements, which include making multiple follow-up visits and filling out question-naires about their pets' symptoms. Once they are accepted into research programs, Brown said, she often marvels at the owners' dedication to completing all the tasks they were asked to perform.

"We once had owners who spent their summers in Colorado, but still flew back with their dog every month to come in for exams," Brown said. "It's pretty amazing what people will do for the sake of their pet, as well as for the sake of moving the science forward."

Breast cancer, perhaps more than any other I had come across in my comparative-oncology travels, seemed to be a powerful mobilizing force for the participants in Sorenmo's mammary tumor research program, many of whom had experienced the disease themselves or knew people who had. Just as the loss of my sister drove me to bring atten-tion to comparative oncology, their breast cancer experi-ences made them passionate about Sorenmo's study.

Sorenmo lost her mother to breast cancer, and a few days before I met her, she learned that her sister had just been diagnosed with the disease. Several of her colleagues were also battling breast cancer or had family members who were, she said. As she looked at her computer screen, which was filled with a collage of photos of the dogs in her research program, Sorenmo told me she felt she just couldn't escape this formidable cancer that was stalking so many women in her life.

"It's scary," said Sorenmo, who was thin and blonde and spoke in a soft Scandinavian accent tinged with urgency and a bit of anger. "It has made me more acutely aware of the importance of this research. We want to move forward faster."

Sorenmo turned her computer screen toward me to show me a photo of a Chihuahua with a tumor so enormous it covered her entire belly. This was Lala, who arrived at Penn from a local rescue group in the spring of 2011, unable to move or rest comfortably. Sorenmo removed the tumor, which was mostly benign. But there was one tiny section that had started to metastasize. Sorenmo's plan was to send the benign and cancerous tissues to Troyanskaya, who would analyze the genes from the two samples and compare them to each other.

"How do you know what to look for?" I asked Sorenmo.

"You don't," she said. "That's why you have to do a complete sequencing of the benign and cancerous tissue — so you can sort out the differences."

Lala didn't need any chemo after her surgery, and she found a new home with Florence Murray, a veterinary technician at Penn who had assisted in Lala's surgery. The day I visited, Murray had brought Lala to work with her, dressing her in a t-shirt to protect the tiny dog from the chill of the clinic's air conditioning. The t-shirt was embla-zoned with a cartoon dog draped in pink ribbon — the logo of Sorenmo's research program.

Murray already had four cats, two dogs, and a tortoise, she told me, but she couldn't resist adding the scruffy tan-and-white Chihuahua to the menagerie.

"She was just as sweet as she could be. She just wanted to be loved and talked to," Murray said. "I kept thinking nobody's going to take her home — people don't go look-ing for a sick dog. I couldn't let her go."

Lala soon became the houschold's alpha dog, Murray said, chasing the cats and climbing on the back of the couch so she could look out the window and bark at vis-itors. Lala was estimated to be twelve years old when she arrived at Penn, and she had never been spayed, so Penn's vets spayed her during the tumor removal surgery. As we played with her in a holding room behind the surgical suite, Murray picked her up, pulled up her t-shirt, and showed me the scar that ran from the top of her sternum down past her lowest rib.

"I'll bet that tumor was half her weight," Murray said. "It's amazing what they can fix." Many Chihuahuas live to eighteen, she added, and as Lala scampered around the room, Murray predicted the dog would live that long, cancer-free.

I wondered whether, like so many of the other partic-ipants in the trial, Murray had a personal experience with breast cancer. She told me she had lost a favorite aunt to the disease, then later witnessed a close friend wage an exhausting battle against it.

"She had breast cancer, then she got cervical cancer and

had to have a hysterectomy," Murray said. "How much can one person go through? I'm hopeful this research will open new possibilities for treatment."

Sorenmo was particularly interested in figuring out what makes breast tumors spread. While she was working in Norway, she started a study of 236 tumors taken from ninety dogs, and later published a paper pointing out the many commonalities between dogs with mammary tumors and women with breast cancer. She noted, for example, that in both species, the risk of malignancy increases with age. Dogs can develop more than eight tumor types in their mammary glands, but the deadliest cancer — the one most likely to spread — is a simple carcinoma that's identical to the most commonly diagnosed breast tumor in women.[10]

But what exactly is happening inside the breast tissue that causes normal cells to become carcinomas? Are genetic mutations transforming benign masses into aggressive cancers? Sorenmo believed that if she could find the answer to that question in mammary tumors, her contribution to cancer research would stretch well beyond breast cancer.

"It's metastasis that kills the cancer patient," she said. "My mom was sixty when she was diagnosed, and she already had metastases. She was dead by sixty-three."

It's true that in virtually all cancers, advancements in surgical techniques have greatly improved patient outcomes — but only if the disease hasn't already spread. Five-year survival rates for women diagnosed with breast cancer prior to metastasis are 93 percent or better, but they fall to 72 percent once the cancer begins to spread.[11] Colon cancer has a 92 percent cure rate in its earliest phase,[12] and early-stage gastric cancer can be successfully beaten 71 percent of the time with surgery to remove the tumor or the entire stomach before metastasis.[13]

When I met Sorenmo, she told me she had to stop enrolling new dogs in the mammary cancer study, because she was struggling to raise the money to continue the research. This surprised me. I figured with all the pink-ribbon promotions and celebrity-filled walkathons, there would be plenty of grants out there for innovative projects aimed at curing breast cancer. And there are.

As of early 2015, the American Cancer Society was devoting $116.1 million in grants to 204 breast cancer research projects — far eclipsing its next most well financed research priority, colorectal cancer, for which it was funding 100 grants worth $56.8 million.[14] Similarly, the National Cancer Institute has devoted more than $550 million annually to breast cancer research each year since 2010. In 2011, the $625 million it spent on breast cancer research was double what it devoted to lung and prostate cancer research.[15] Even the National Football League is giving money to breast cancer research — its Crucial Catch program donates $1 million every year from the proceeds of selling pink football gear online and at games.[16]

I asked Sorenmo why she couldn't find just one deep-pocketed donor among all those organizations to keep her study alive.

"We've tried. We haven't been successful," Sorenmo said. "When they comment on our proposals, they tell us they don't understand why we would want to study dogs."

While Sorenmo worked to secure more research funding,

she continued to care for the dogs who had already been treated through the program. The day I was there, she had scheduled a follow-up exam of Lady, a thirteen-year-old shepherd–husky mix, who came into the mammary tumor program through Faith's Hope, a Philadelphia animal rescue group.

Rosemary Sariego, who runs Faith's Hope, had found the dog neglected and whimpering in her owners' backyard, where she was kept day and night regardless of the weather. Sariego called the SPCA, which picked up Lady and brought her to the shelter, where a vet discovered she had an infected uterus and several mammary tumors. Despite her beautiful black-and-brown coat and unusual blue eyes, the shelter deemed Lady to be an unlikely candidate for adoption because of her advanced age and poor health.

The SPCA put Lady on the schedule to be euthanized. So Sariego took her home, found a family to adopt her, then called up Sorenmo and asked if she would take the dog into the mammary tumor program. Some of Lady's tumors were metastatic, Sorenmo told me, but after she removed all the carcinomas, the dog was fine.

Faith's Hope brought four more dogs with mammary cancer to Sorenmo's clinic. Among them was Rini, a Shih Tzu mix with cancerous tumors in half her mammary glands, all of which were removed for the study. Sariego adopted Rini herself. When I spoke to Sariego two years later, the black-and-white lapdog with a raccoon-like face was healthy, active, and still cancer-free.

"These dogs didn't have a chance," Sariego said. "Now they'll get care for the rest of their lives. It's a godsend, and they're helping human research."

In addition to appealing to traditional cancer research groups for funding, Sorenmo and Troyanskaya approached comparative oncology foundations, most of which were started by people who had lost their dogs to cancer. In January 2012, they were thrilled to learn they had received a $50,000 grant from 2 Million Dogs (later renamed Puppy Up), a foundation that was founded in 2008 by Luke Robinson, who walked two thousand miles from Austin to Boston to raise money for comparative oncology research. Robinson, who lost his Great Pyrenees to osteosarcoma, met Sorenmo when he was walking through Philadelphia. The grant for the mammary tumor research was the first awarded by his foundation.

Armed with the new money, Sorenmo selected samples she had collected from seventeen dogs. Each of the dogs had at least one benign mass and one malignant tumor. She sent the samples to Troyanskaya, who isolated and analyzed the RNA in each sample. RNA (ribonucleic acid) analysis allows scientists to determine which genes are turned on or off or expressed at high and low levels in various scenarios. Abnormalities in gene expression — the process by which the body's cells take the information encoded in genes and turn it into something functional, like a protein — drive many cancers. Troyanskaya would look for changes that occurred as the tumors progressed from benign to malignant.

Troyanskaya planned to compare her findings to data generated from gene expression studies of human breast cancer samples. She expected to find correlations between dog and human, but she hoped that the benign and malignant samples from the dogs would help her identify the signals that govern the progression of breast cancer.

"What we really hope is to come up with a set of genes that might be predictive," Troyanskaya told me when I reached her by phone to get her take on the research. "That way, we'd be able to actually look at a benign tumor and say whether this tumor has the potential to become malignant."

If they could scrape up more funding, Troyanskaya said, they would be able to analyze protein expression in the canine tumor samples. That would not only shed more light on gene activity in breast cancer, it would also point to potential cures.

"At the very least we would get a better molecular understanding of what's happening when these cancers develop," Troyanskaya said. "And potentially we'll get better targets for therapy."

In addition to collaborating with Troyanskaya at Princeton, Sorenmo hoped to team up with oncologists at Penn's Abramson Cancer Center, which had already worked with the veterinary school on a comparative lymphoma study.

Sorenmo said that, with the memory of her mother's unsuccessful fight against breast cancer still raw, she had felt camaraderie with all the dogs who were fighting the disease and the pet owners like Mildred Edmond who shared her passion for finding a cure. She clicked through more photos of dogs, pausing at Cali's.

"There have been a lot of relationships that have formed through this program," she said. "These dogs somehow appeal to people who have a history themselves of hardship. The fact that Mildred had breast cancer herself and the two of them found each other . . . Cali has become the poster child for everything we want to do with this program."

Cali had settled into a life of sunbathing and enjoying hand-fed soft biscuits, which she gnawed on with the sole fang left in her bottom jaw — a visible quirk that prompted Edmond to nickname her Snaggle Tooth. Edmond and Cali returned to Penn yearly for checkups.

The day before I met Edmond, she had been to a follow-up appointment with the surgeon who removed her breast tumor. Edmond's tumor had not tested positive for mutations or other characteristics that could be addressed by targeted drugs, so her doctors had no choice but to rely on surgery and old chemo regimens.

I asked her if she ever thought about her cancer coming back.

"I get worried. Like yesterday, the surgeon kept pushing on this one side. When they stay too long at one spot it makes me nervous," said Edmond, who worked at a plumbing supply shop near her home. "But it was just calcification. I've had my mammograms, and nothing has changed."

Edmond was just as vigilant about keeping Cali healthy as she was about checking her own breasts regularly.

"I run my fingers around her belly, too, to make sure there are no more lumps."

Edmond had struck an agreement with Penn's vet school that, after Cali died, she would donate the dog's body to the study, so veterinarians there could continue to learn from her cancer experience.

"She's going to be a big help to the study," Edmond said, "living or not."

Chapter 7

From iPods to Cowpox:
Offbeat Attacks against Solid Tumors

A physician in Ann Arbor, Michigan, named George Dock was treating a forty-two-year-old woman for leukemia when she came down with a bad case of the flu. Much to Dock's surprise, the patient's cancerous liver and spleen, which had been greatly enlarged by the disease, returned to their normal sizes. Her white blood cells — the immune cells that grow out of control in patients with leukemia and other blood-born cancers — began to vanish, dropping sevenfold in the days following her bout with the virus. She enjoyed a short remission from her cancer.

Dock later wrote a paper about the case, strongly urging the medical community to examine whether the answer to treating cancer lies in other diseases.[1]

That was in 1896 — a full thirty-seven years before scientists were even able to classify influenza as a virus. And the medical journals continued to publish report after report of cancer patients whose disease disappeared after they were struck by another illness, usually the flu or the measles or something else that would later prove to be a virus.

By the 1950s, the scientific community fully understood many of the characteristics that made viruses different from other microbes, most notably their ability to invade just about any cell in the body and replicate inside of it, causing everything from mild illnesses like the common cold to crippling and sometimes deadly plagues, such as polio and smallpox. This discovery had oncology researchers all over the world harkening back to Dock's leukemia patient and the other virus-stricken cancer patients whose remarkable — albeit brief — remissions were still being reported in medical journals. They began trying to turn viruses into cancer drugs and tested them on patients.

Nothing worked. The viruses were either too weak to wage an effective attack against tumors or they were so strong they put patients at risk of dying from a lethal immune response, not to the cancer but to the viruses themselves. By the end of the 1970s, the search for cancer-killing viruses was all but abandoned.[2]

Two decades later, Aladár Szalay, a Hungarian-born molecular geneticist, started a biotech company in San Diego with the intention of developing virus-based drugs to treat a range of solid tumors. From day one, Szalay believed pet dogs with cancer would help him resurrect the field of virotherapy.

By this time, genetic engineering had evolved to the point where scientists could tweak the viruses — removing links from their DNA chains, or adding links to them. Such genetic changes improved the ability of the viruses to find and kill cancer cells, while at the same time ensuring healthy cells would be spared. Szalay and others working in the field believed these advances would prevent the dangerous immune storms that had foiled so many past virotherapies.

Genelux's lead drug was a genetically modified form of vaccinia, more commonly known as cowpox. This is the same virus that is the basis of the smallpox vaccine, which was given to hundreds of millions of people around the world starting in 1798 and ending in 1980, when the World Health Organization declared the disease eradicated.[3] Vaccinia had proven so safe in people that when virotherapy was revived, oncologists identified it early on as a prime candidate for cancer drug development.

Vaccination and virotherapy are similar in that they both use attenuated viruses to activate the immune system. But that's where the similarities end. In response to vaccination, the immune system produces antibodies, which protect the patient against the virus for many years to come. In virotherapy against cancer, on the other hand, the virus itself is the weapon — targeting and invading cancer cells, replicating inside them, and ultimately killing them.[4]

Genelux's vaccinia technology had two distinct features. First, the virus was constructed with transgenes — synthesized genetic materials that boosted its ability to home in on specific types of solid tumors. Second, the virus carried a light-emitting gene, which churned out a protein called luciferase. When I met him, Szalay explained that luciferase causes the virus to glow in the dark, allowing physicians to track its activity in patients using standard imaging devices, like MRI machines. When injected into the bloodstream, the theory was, vaccinia would replicate inside cells, kill them, then travel to other cancer cells, chipping away at the tumor until it was gone.

In June 2012, Genelux issued a press release announcing it was recruiting dogs for a study of an experimental drug called V-VETI, a genetically modified form of cowpox that was similar to a cancer therapy Genelux was developing for people.[5] Szalay selected Gregory Ogilvie, director of the Angel Care Cancer Center at California Veterinary Specialists in San Diego, to run the dog trial. Ogilvie was a former Colorado State University faculty member with a bit of a reputation for supporting off-beat, experimental approaches to treating cancer.

It's rare for a company to broadcast an animal trial with a press release — drug-developers often shroud such research in secrecy to avoid raising the hackles of animal-rights groups — but when I sat down with Szalay in his office a few months later, on a rare sweltering day for San Diego, he told me he wanted the world to understand that his scientists were proud of the work they were doing to benefit both people and pets with cancer.

Szalay told me that he had fond memories of growing up with dogs on a farm in a small village of Hungary called Bogyiszló. His family had a Hungarian Puli, a herding dog with dreadlock-like cords — a distinctive coat that prompts some dog show commentators to jokingly call the canine a walking mop. Szalay spent many hours playing with the dog, who pulled him through the snow on makeshift sled, he recalled. Szalay's two grown daughters had dogs, he told me. But in a period of just two years, three of the four dogs owned by his daughters' families died of cancer, instilling in Szalay a passion to make a contribution to veterinary medicine.

"We should all come to the realization that animals also need our help and should not just be tools for preparing or improving human drugs," Szalay said. "I'm convinced of this fact."

Szalay has been fascinated with genetic engineering since the mid-1980s, when he was earning his Ph.D. at Cornell University. He was part of a team that figured out how to monitor genes in live cells by using luciferase to get them to light up. The discovery became the basis of Genelux, and Szalay was still so excited about the science that as soon as I sat down in the company's conference room, he spoke about it for seventeen minutes straight, stopping only to ask an assistant to bring a large fan to back up the company's faltering air conditioning.

Szalay beamed a slide onto a movie screen and pointed excitedly at photos of one of Genelux's glowing viruses invading a cancer cell and then replicating inside it.

"Fourteen days after injection, the tumor shrinks, the light is there and the virus material is enormous," he said. "After twenty-eight days, the tumor is smaller, and the light is still there," which showed that the virus was still replicating inside the tumor, he explained.

"After fifty-six days, lo and behold, the light is gone," Szalay said with such giddiness it was almost as if he were discovering the virus's talents for the first time.

"The tumor is gone."

The first dog enrolled in Genelux's vaccinia trial was a fourteen-year-old terrier mix named Chance. The energetic, thirty-pound black dog with white paws, legs, and eyebrows had a tumor under his tail, and his owner, Ken Willcut, didn't have any good treatment options. Surgery to remove the tumor would have cost at least $2,000 — far more than Willcut, a sales representative for Coca-Cola, thought he could afford. And he was afraid such a drastic treatment would hamper Chance's ability to enjoy being a dog.

"He's got so much life in him," Willcut told me shortly after Chance entered the Genelux trial. "He's still bouncing off the walls like terriers do. I just wanted to be able to maintain his quality of life."

Willcut first met Chance at the local shelter near his home in Lake Elsinore, California, which had put the puppy on its list to be euthanized. They told Willcut they had found him in a dumpster.

Willcut returned to the shelter the following day, only to discover a staff member was already in the dog's kennel preparing the lethal injection. Willcut adopted the dog and named him Last Chance, because he knew he had given the terrier a last chance at life.

Chance saw Willcut pass one milestone after another, including his marriage and the birth of his daughter. The dog quickly adjusted to all the changes, embracing each new family member, which included a rescued Chihuahua named Lupe. Chance was Willcut's constant companion, accompanying him on camping and motorcycling trips, thrilled just to be there, wherever *there* might be.

When Gregory Ogilvie met Chance, he thought the dog's name was apropos. The dog, after all, was giving the world a chance to find out if a new type of virotherapy had the potential to treat cancer. Ogilvie and his staff gave Chance injections of v-veti weekly for several months, meticulously measuring the tumor each week. It seemed to be shrinking, and Chance suffered no side effects from the treatment.

Ogilvie was taking me on a walking tour of his cancer clinic in Carlsbad, California, regaling me with stories about Genelux's dog trial and other research he was involved in, when he opened a cabinet full of pill bottles and medical instruments and pulled out a purple iPod Nano with a plastic tube sticking out of it.

Ogilvie handed the iPod to me and explained that he was also working with a nearby company named Nativis, which was using the music player to test its theory that energy fields emitted by cancer drugs might be more effective at treating cancer than the drugs themselves. Nativis was working on a Nano-inspired device that was designed to separate the healing part of the medicine from its more toxic elements and then turn the positive energy into an audio file that could be recorded and subsequently emitted to patients. Ogilvie began enrolling pet dogs into a trial of an early version Nativis's technology — delivered by the Nano — around the same time he launched the Genelux trial.

"It's literally quantum physics," Ogilvie said of Nativis's idea. "We call it the Black Eyed Peas therapy."

I laughed nervously at Ogilvie's joke, as I fiddled with the plastic tube that purportedly transformed the music player into a therapy-delivery device. I was trying hard to contain the skepticism I had honed during my years covering the biotechnology industry. An iPod as a device to cure cancer? And it's not the drug being delivered, but its energy? This seemed more like sci-fi than a serious medical pursuit.

Then Ogilvie told me about the first dog to participate in the trial of the experimental product. The dog had a tumor on her paw, Ogilvie said, but because she was pregnant, it wasn't safe for her to receive chemo. So Ogilvie tried the experimental technology.

"The big tumor on the paw disappeared," Ogilvie said. "The dog then had her pups and nursed the pups. To the best of our knowledge, she is still doing well." If the other dogs in the trial responded that well, Ogilvie said, Nativis would try the device in people.

Ogilvie had spent much of his twenty-five-year career looking for alternatives to chemotherapy and radiation — new gizmos or vitamins or nutritional regimens that might combat the disease without causing untoward side effects. He had investigated dietary fatty acids, for example, to see if they would delay relapse in patients who had already been treated successfully with standard cancer drugs. He also participated in some of the early dog trials of MTP-PE — the drug that Denver Children's Hospital physicians had used on young Emily Brown. The MTP-PE experience, he said, taught him the value of searching for cures along the far fringes of traditional medicine.

"That work showed that if you stimulate the immune system you can defeat cancer," said Ogilvie, who escorted me from the clinic's operating suite to a room at the back of the clinic, with soft couches and a secluded feel. This was where some clients chose to spend their last moments with their gravely ill pets, he told me. Then he quietly explained why he was so open to trying therapies that other scientists might write off as too bizarre.

"One of the ways in which we can get rid of cancer is with chemotherapy, but there seems to be a wall," Ogilvie said. "We can get patients to a certain point, but how can we go beyond that? Cancer occurs when our immune systems fail us. We can use science and technology to overcome that."

While working as a full-time veterinarian, Ogilvie was also serving as the director of veterinary medicine at the University of California at San Diego. This was an odd faculty appointment, as the university did not even have a veterinary school. Ogilvie's boss at UCSD, Arno James Mundt, told me that with all the advances in comparative oncology, it just made sense for UCSD to add an animal doctor to the faculty.

"I thought if I put a lot of bright people together and pressed 'mix,' great things would happen," Mundt said. "When you're looking at novel agents like viruses, it's natural to study them in dogs because they have so many interesting parallels to humans. It's just exciting."

Genelux had already been working with UCSD on perfecting its virus technology when Mundt introduced Szalay to Ogilvie. The CEO and the veterinarian hit it off.

Szalay had tried for years to persuade veterinarians at the University of Hanover in Germany to launch a trial of Genelux's technology in pet dogs, to no avail. Without hesitation, Ogilvie agreed to do the trial.

"I knew the virus was safe — it's been around for a very long time and has a distinguished career of saving millions from infectious disease," Ogilvie said. "I became extraordinarily excited about the potential of finding out if this could provide an innovative approach to conquering cancer."

Chance did well on the v-VETI at first. But one day in late 2012, after Chance had finished the twelve-week course of the experimental drug, Willcut noticed the dog was struggling to walk. He figured the effects of the tumor and Chance's advanced age had become too much for the dog to endure. He knew it was time to say goodbye.

"I just think we caught the tumor too late," Willcut said, adding that he never regretted the decision to enter the Genelux trial with Chance. "The whole point was to help in any way we could. As much as he liked to be around people, we hoped he could give them a little more of a gift, beyond just his personality."

———

While Ogilvie and Szalay were laboring to prove vaccinia's value as a cancer treatment, veterinarians around the world were using genetic engineering to create all sorts of other immunological weapons against the disease — and enlisting dogs to help prove they could work.

At the University of Minnesota, for example, veterinarians were creating and testing personalized vaccines against glioblastoma, a common and deadly form of brain cancer. They removed parts of the tumors from dogs with the disease, then used each dog's own cancer cells to make the vaccine, which was then injected back into the patient. The theory was that each dog's immune system would identify the cancer as foreign and go on an attack against what remained of the tumor. The university's medical school was testing a similar approach in people.[6]

Meanwhile several research groups were identifying canine viruses that bore similarities to human viruses, and then studying them to see if they might be effective against cancer.[7] For example, when Cheryl London was at UC Davis, she and her colleagues investigated canine distemper virus as a possible treatment for lymphoma. Distemper is part of a family known as Morbilliviruses, which also include human measles. When Morbilliviruses infect their victims, they trigger a variety of reactions, including lymphopenia, which is a reduction in some white blood cells — the very cells that grow out of control in patients with lymphoma. That's why Morbilliviruses have long been of interest to virotherapy researchers.

In the UC Davis study, veterinarians took tumor samples from dogs with lymphoma, isolated the cancer cells and then infected the cells with an attenuated version of the distemper virus. Using genetic sequencing, they showed that within two days, the cancer cells began the process of apoptosis — the systematic cell suicide that so many cancer treatments were designed to stimulate. In their 2005 paper describing the experiment, London and her colleagues suggested that the distemper virus be studied as a possible treatment for canine lymphoma, "with the intention that information gained from these studies will have direct applicability to the future treatment of human patients with non–Hodgkin's lymphoma."[8]

In Brazil, a team of scientists were curious to see if canine distemper virus could be effective against cancers that were traditionally resistant to apoptosis. So they took a population of human cervical cancer cells and infected them with distemper. They discovered that the virus activated a protein called executioner caspase-3, which is a key promoter of cell death, as its name indicates. The cancerous cells began to die.[9]

By 2013, Genelux found itself in a race with scientists at dozens of biotech companies and academic researchers who had all found innovative ways to engineer human viruses to train them to attack cancer. Vaccinia remained a popular tool, but it was far from the only virus of interest. Some scientists were working with measles, others with the herpes virus, and still others with a family of microorganisms known as reoviruses, which are relatively common viruses that cause mostly mild intestinal and respiratory illnesses in humans.

The entire field of virotherapy got a boost in late 2013, when the world's largest biotech company, Amgen, in Thousand Oaks, California, released a string of positive clinical trial results on TVEC, its engineered herpes virus, which it was testing on melanoma. Amgen acquired the inventor of TVEC (short for talimogene laherparepvec),

BioVex, in 2011, when the drug was still in the early stages of development, for a remarkable $1 billion — a risky bet at the time, considering virotherapy's checkered past.

The scientists who originally engineered TVEC built into the virus the ability to churn out a protein called GM-CSF (granulocyte-macrophage colony-stimulating factor). GM-CSF was similar to MTP-PE in that it helped the immune system fight cancer. GM-CSF's particular talent was to lure immune-boosting white cells into tumors. Those cells then accelerated the virus's cancer-killing activity.

In September 2013, Amgen revealed that 19 percent of melanoma patients in a late-stage clinical trial who received TVEC had a durable response — meaning their cancer was under control for a significant length of time — whereas only 1 percent of patients who just took GM-CSF saw this kind of improvement. In 68 percent of patients who responded to TVEC, the positive effect lasted nine months or more.[10] Amgen filed for FDA approval in 2014.

Genelux, having scraped together only a few million dollars in funding from private investors, was progressing much more slowly on its virotherapy research than its rivals were. The company began a small trial of its drug in German patients in April 2012, and it reported somewhat positive results in a rare cancer that affects the lining of the peritoneal cavity.[11] Then Genelux treated a handful of patients at UCSD and Memorial Sloan Kettering Cancer Center in New York. But thousands more patients would need to be exposed to the newfangled viruses, and then tracked for years, to make sure there were no untoward circumstances to this new mode of therapy.

One feature of viruses that makes them so attractive as cancer remedies, Szalay told me, is that they seem to work against so many different types of tumors. Viruses generally don't discriminate — they treat any cancer cell, it seems, as an enemy. Genelux held human trials in no less than a half-dozen cancers, including prostate cancer, mesothelioma, and head and neck tumors. After the initial veterinary trial at Ogilvie's clinic, Genelux continued to develop V-VETI, and was seeing potential for the drug in a range of tumor types, including osteosarcoma, mammary cancer, and mast cell tumors.

Szalay wasn't sure when he would see his or any other company's virotherapy on the market, but he knew he had to keep trying. He still had the grand dream of attaching other therapies to his viruses to make them even more potent, such as anti-angiogenic drugs to cut off the blood supply to tumors.

"The opportunity to use the virus not just as a tumor killer, but also an additional drug-delivery system, is enormous," he said. "In animals, too."

Shortly after I learned about virotherapy during my trip to San Diego, I visited my parents and asked to copy the e-mails we all received from Beth during her cancer battle. My mother had saved them all in a folder with the sad title "Beth's condition." After my sister died, in the grips of grief, I had deleted most of those e-mails from my own computer.

At the time, I wanted to erase all the bad memories. But now, as dogs had revived my hope in cancer research, I felt better prepared to relive the cycle of hope and disappointment that marked that terrible year.

One by one, I forwarded them to myself — all 127 e-mails. They sat unopened in my e-mail inbox for months, until I finally worked up the nerve to relive all the painful memories.

One of the first e-mails we received came a few weeks after the diagnosis, when we learned of the chemo regimen Beth's oncologist, Dan Aderka, had selected. The cocktail included three of the oldest cancer drugs around: epirubicin, on the market in the U.S. since 1999,[12] cisplatin, first approved in 1978,[13] and the granddaddy of them all, fluorouracil (5-FU), which has been used in cancer treatment since 1962.[14]

Then Beth learned her insurance company would allow Aderka to prescribe a new drug in place of 5-FU — a chemo pill she could take at home, instead of having to get it intravenously in the hospital along with the other two. This seemed like good news to me. The pill had been on the market for twelve years but had just been shown to be effective in gastric cancer. This new medicine just had to be better than that ancient 5 FU, I convinced myself.

I told my sister that the chemo pill had been developed partly with the aim of reducing the toxic side effects of cancer treatment. I felt hope. I heard hope in my sister's voice when she told me her nurses had predicted she wouldn't lose her hair.

"I'm dreaming about you every night, but they've all been hopeful dreams," I wrote to Beth on the eve of her first treatment.

"I'm glad to get going with it," she responded. "I'll try to be in touch when I'm feeling better in between treatments."

But there was no feeling better. Despite her nurses' prediction, Beth lost her hair. She was so sick she couldn't talk on the phone or sit at her computer to write even the briefest of e-mails. Beth's stomach tumor did respond to the treatment — shrinking so dramatically, in fact, that her oncologists briefly contemplated whether they had got her diagnosis wrong. Perhaps the cancer had started somewhere else, they thought, and the stomach tumor was merely an outgrowth of a different type of cancer that responds more favorably to chemo than gastric tumors typically do.

Their hope, and our hope, was fleeting, however. When Beth's surgeons went in to remove what was left of the stomach tumor, they discovered the cancer had spread much more than they originally thought.

It was not until after her death that I was able to accept the truth about that chemo pill: There was little new about it except for the pill itself. The medicine inside the pill transformed into 5-FU as soon as it entered the patient's bloodstream. Was this a more convenient way to receive chemo than having to travel to a clinic and get hooked up to an IV system? Perhaps. But that pill was nothing more than a fifty-year-old medicine in a shiny new package.

The pursuit of new approaches to treating cancer is a centuries-old quest marked by dead ends, crushed expectations, and billions of dollars poured into ideas that ultimately prove useless. For patients and their families, though, the promise of something new is irresistible. New is a potential cure. New is a chance to live. I had been clutching onto the promise inherent in a new drug, but it really held no such promise.

When I met the scientists and veterinarians working to resurrect the field of virotherapy, I was inspired by their efforts to take a 150-year-old idea and infuse it with advanced technology that might transform the common virus into something truly new, truly revolutionary. George Dock and his leukemia patient were not forgotten. The inkling that viruses may cure cancer had been revived, recharged with the promise of genetic engineering, and reclaimed by people who understood that when you're fighting the smartest foe in medicine, you should never abandon any new idea if you have the chance to improve upon it.

"I always say, 'If you keep your eyes open, you'll see miracles every day,'" Ogilvie told me. And, he added, when it comes to cancer research, the most important quality was simple: "You can't let anyone stand in your way."

As I was leaving Genelux, Szalay told me a story about one of his granddaughters, who once had a dream of becoming a veterinarian. But after she lost a favorite dog to cancer, she changed her mind — a decision that broke her grandpa's heart.

"I asked her, 'What happened?'" Szalay said. "She started to cry and said, 'I do not want to put down people's loved ones. This should not be my job.'"

Szalay made a vow to his granddaughter, telling her that if she became a veterinary oncologist, he would help her build an animal hospital right next door to a children's cancer clinic. He promised her that someday there would be many new treatments that would help save lives in her clinic — and in the one next door, too.

"Then," Szalay told the little girl, "you can help dogs *and* children."

Chapter 8
The Feline Connection

In the summer of 2014, veterinarians at the University of Guelph's Ontario Veterinary College began looking for house cats to help them answer a tantalizing question: Could a virus that originates in Brazilian sand flies be transformed into a cure for some cancers? J. Paul Woods, professor of internal medicine oncology at the Canadian college, had been waiting more than three years to start the trial, and when I spoke to him late that summer, he had just signed up the first of what he hoped would be thirty feline participants.

"Whenever someone called wanting to enroll, before, we had to say, 'I'm sorry, I can't help your cat. The feds will not let us open the trial,'" Woods said. "We just got our license from the federal government. We are so excited to finally be starting."

The experimental virus's journey from Brazilian insect to Canadian cat was a case study in frustration, learning, and remarkable perseverance. The project started at McMaster University in Hamilton, Ontario, where a group of scientists had been studying oncolytic viruses — those that preferentially target cancer cells — since the late 1990s. Through a process called bioprospecting they collected viruses from all over the world, not just from insects, but from reptiles, mammals, and birds, too.

They introduced each virus to tumor cells and observed what happened under a microscope, and they were struck by the potential of the Brazilian virus, named Maraba after the region where it was first isolated in the 1980s. Maraba stood out as a superpower of oncolytic villains, said Brian Lichty, associate professor of pathology and molecular medicine at the McMaster Immunology Research Centre.

"It loves to grow in tumor cells and destroy them," he said.

But that wasn't all the virus could offer. It also has a tiny genome, which means it can replicate rapidly. But it can only replicate in a cell's cytoplasm, the material that surrounds but is outside the nucleus, which means it can't reach and mutate its host's genome and cause untoward side effects, Lichty said. And there doesn't seem to be any pre-existing immunity to the virus that would need to be overcome in either cats or people.

Lichty and his research team were aware of other oncolytic viruses that were being developed around the world, but they saw something else that made Maraba distinctive — something they believed would set their project apart from all the others. The virus could be engineered to leave behind specific cancer-killing antigens, which would work indefinitely to prevent the cancer from coming back.

"We layered extra technology onto this so it would be like any other vaccine," Lichty said. "For a week or so It destroys the tumors, but then it continues the attack, cleaning up what was missed and preventing relapse."

The engineered virus worked in mouse models, but that wasn't good enough for Lichty. He thought the virus held great potential for treating the most aggressive form of breast cancer in women. And having grown up on a farm surrounded by barn cats, he immediately thought of feline mammary cancer as a perfect model of the human disease.

In one significant way cats are even better models for breast cancer than dogs are. Breast cancer is the third most common feline cancer.[1] Cats are particularly prone to a type of mammary tumor that's similar to one that afflicts women and has proven to be stubborn to treat. But while dogs can often be cured with surgery and chemotherapy, mammary cancer in cats is not so easy to conquer. That's because about 90 percent of mammary tumors in cats are malignant.[2]

"I don't have anything that I know works well in cats," Woods said. "If I had a novel therapy that I knew was working, we'd move so much further ahead."

For Woods, running the cat study marked an important milestone in the University of Guelph's emergence as a major comparative oncology center. Born in Canada, Woods got his veterinary degree at the University of Guelph. He completed his oncology fellowship at Colorado State University in 2004 then returned to Canada with the goal of building a comprehensive veterinary cancer center like the one he trained at in Fort Collins.

Initially, the university's veterinary oncology service resided within the Ontario Veterinary College, which was founded in 1862, making it the oldest continuously operating vet school in North America.[3] In 2007, Woods helped to launch the Institute for Comparative Cancer Investigation at the university — the first research center devoted to comparative oncology in Canada. In late 2012, the college opened a new hospital dedicated exclusively to treating pets with cancer and to running oncology clinical trials, many of which are comparative. The university became the only Canadian member of the National Cancer Institute's United States–based Comparative Oncology Trials Consortium.

The institute was running as many as ten comparative trials simultaneously, Woods said, but the oncolytic virus research was among the first to include cats. He was optimistic he'd find plenty of cat owners willing to take a chance on the exotic virus-based therapy; the college, after all, is situated in southern Ontario, with ten million Canadians and Americans living within a hundred miles of the vet school.

Finding the cats that would be the most suitable for the trial, however, would be far from a simple task. Cats are not called upon to participate in comparative oncology trials nearly as often as dogs are, for a variety of reasons, not the least of which is their famously independent personality.

Being involved in a clinical trial presents challenges that not everyone can handle, regardless of whether the patient has two legs or four. Trial participants must submit to frequent poking, prodding, and analyzing of every little symptom that arises during the study period. Unlike dogs — who will do just about anything for a treat or a toss of a ball   cats generally demand to be treated on their own terms. That can be a problem.

"Some cats can't even handle the car ride to the clinic," Woods said. "We're trying to increase their quality of life, but if they're that stressed out, it's just not going to work."

Woods and the other veterinarians I met told me that another reason for the lack of feline comparative trials is that they just don't see as many cases of cancer in cats as they see in dogs. And the cancers that cats do get are often quite different from the types of tumors that people get.

Breast cancer is one notable exception. Many mammary tumors in cats, Lichty explained to me, are almost identical to triple-negative human breast cancer, so called because the tumor does not express the genes for estrogen receptor, progesterone receptor, or HER2. That makes it resistant to most available therapies. This was starkly illustrated in a study of more than fifty thousand women listed in the California Cancer Registry, which found that the five-year survival rate for patients with triple-negative breast cancer was 77 percent, versus 93 percent for those suffering from other forms of the disease.[4]

"The feline disease represents the worst-case scenario in the human disease," Lichty said, adding that if a treatment or a cure could be devised, it would be "an easily applied therapy for cats, and for women, who also don't have great options."

Lichty and Woods made such a strong case for the value of the cat trial that the Canadian Breast Cancer Foundation gave them a grant to fund the study. Persuading the Canadian government that the trial was a good idea was much more difficult, however. The organization in charge of the approval was the Canadian Food Inspection Agency (CFIA), Canada's equivalent of the USDA, which as far as Lichty could tell had never been asked to approve a trial of a therapeutic virus in domestic animals.

"The first obstacle was ignorance. Nobody could tell me what I needed to do to get the permit," Lichty recalled.

After the CFIA reviewed the trial plan, the agency told Lichty's team that they would have to first test the virus in six healthy lab cats — a step Lichty had been hoping to avoid. The agency was concerned about the virus "shedding," or inadvertently being released into the environment, where it might infect other animals, plants, or people. CFIA officials wanted to see what would happen when the therapy was administered in a controlled environment first, before accepting the risk of pet cats getting treated with a little-understood viral vaccine and then returning home to their families. The lab cats wouldn't be given cancer, as the rodents used in preclinical cancer trials often are, but Lichty was still bothered that the trial was required.

"One of my reasons to start doing comparative oncology trials was to stop using research animals," Lichty said. "This forced me to do something that was the opposite of my intention. But there was no way around it."

Fortunately Lichty and Woods were able to show that the virus didn't shed, nor did it cause any toxic effects to the healthy cats. All six were unscathed by the end of the trial, and the researchers got the go-ahead from CFIA to start studying the virus in pet cats.

Woods' plan was to inject the engineered Maraba virus into each cat who was enrolled, perform surgery to remove the tumors, then treat the cats with the virus again. Lichty's team would inspect the samples to determine how the virus was interacting with the cancerous cells. Then the cats would be tracked and called in for periodic blood tests, which would show whether the vaccine was still at work, fending off a recurrence of the cancer.

"We will follow them theoretically for the rest of their lives," Woods said. "If it works, that could be years."

———

When I started delving into comparative oncology, I didn't intend to include cats in my research. Then, in November 2013, I attended the Zoobiquity conference at Rockefeller University in New York — a regular gathering of veterinarians and human health professionals that was inspired by the 2012 book of the same name. This version of the conference included case studies of three very different patients facing similar diagnoses of breast cancer. One was a post-menopausal woman. The second was an eleven-year-old domestic short-haired cat named Magik. And the third was Rika, a fifteen-year-old Siberian tiger at the Bronx Zoo.

Oncologist Larry Norton of Memorial Sloan Kettering discussed the challenges he confronted treating his patients, and the difficult choices many of his patients faced between lumpectomy and mastectomy, for example, or hormonal therapy and chemotherapy. After listening to presentations from two veterinarians who joined him on stage, he told the audience he believed cats could be just as valuable as dogs in helping to solve the so-far insurmountable obstacles to breast cancer prevention and treatment.

After the conference, I asked *Zoobiquity* co-author and the conference's co-chair, physician Barbara Natterson-Horowitz, whether she thought technology had advanced to the point where observations made in animals and people could be combined with genomic data, generating insights that could improve the prevention and treatment of certain cancers.

"Definitely," replied Natterson-Horowitz, a professor of medicine at the University of California at Los Angeles. "Take the case of breast cancer. Zoo veterinarians know that big cats, like lions and tigers and jaguars, who are treated with progestin have an elevated incidence of breast cancer. And actually jaguars have an elevated risk of breast and ovarian cancer, which may be associated with the genetic mutation BRCA."

The effort to improve cancer prevention and treatment, therefore, could benefit from studying the risks that cats and people share, such as genetic predispositions, and exposure to synthetic hormones and other drugs, she said.

"We can look where breast cancer is and get some important information about human breast cancer and some ideas for how to study the problem," she said. "We can also learn from where breast cancer isn't."

I appreciated what Natterson was telling me about the value of cats in medical research. People often classify themselves as dog people *or* cat people, but I have always been a dog *and* cat lover. My love affair with cats started in the first grade, when I was walking home from school, and a white alley cat trotted up behind me. She came right up to the front door, but I couldn't let her in because my dad was allergic to cats. So I ran inside, grabbed one of our dog's Gaines-Burgers — pressed pseudo-meat patties that were popular in the 1970s — mashed it up into a bowl and brought it back outside.

The cat, whom I uncreatively named Kitty, wasn't fazed that I was feeding her dog food. She came back each afternoon, happy to eat whatever leftovers or dog kibble I had for her, and stuck around long enough for me to spend a few minutes stroking her soft, snow-colored coat. Kitty remained outside, though eventually we did buy her Meow Mix and took her to the vet for essential vaccines.

During the day, the desert landscape near our home in Tucson, Arizona, was Kitty's playground, but every afternoon she showed up at our house, looking for me. Kitty will always have a special place in my memory, because while our dogs were family pets, the cat was most definitely mine. She taught me how to be responsible for another living creature, and she showed me that it's okay to be independent, as long as you have someone to rely on when you need help, or even just a cuddle.

Besides their inherent uncooperativeness, cats have played less of a role in comparative oncology than dogs because not as much is known about the feline genome. In 2007, two years after sequencing the dog genome, scientists at the Broad Institute took a major step toward filling that knowledge gap. They published the sequenced genome of an Abyssinian cat named Cinnamon,[5] who had neon green eyes, giant ears, and a coat that matched the color of the spice for which she was named. Then they performed a preliminary analysis, which was not quite as detailed as what they had done for the dog genome but did provide some clues to the potential value of cats in medical research.

One important surprise, said the Broad's scientific director, Kerstin Lindblad-Toh, was the revelation that cats are genetically more similar to people than are mice. Mice should be more like us, she explained, but they have evolved much more quickly than other species have. That has caused them to pull further away from people on the genomic tree, while cats (and, for that matter, dogs) have stayed more in step with us.

In addition to being prone to some of the same cancers, humans and cats share a susceptibility to about forty diseases, including some forms of diabetes, cardiomyopathy, and lupus.[6] And the feline immunodeficiency virus is considered to be the most realistic naturally occurring model of AIDS.

Cats have proven to be especially valuable in advancing the understanding of infectious diseases, as well as the possible role of those illnesses in causing cancer. In 1964, Scottish scientists discovered that a retrovirus caused feline leukemia. They assumed the virus, dubbed feline leukemia virus (FeLV), was inherited.[7]

A few years later, a woman living in Boston walked into the Angel Animal Medical Center looking for help for her thirty-five cats, who lived with her in a one-bedroom apartment. A young veterinarian named Susan Cotter spotted an opportunity in that herd of cats to better understand how exactly FeLV behaved, and if, in fact, it was truly passed down from cat to kitten.

"One day her cats started getting leukemia," recalled Cotter, a professor emeritus at the Cummings School of Veterinary Medicine at Tufts University. "All of her cats were essentially unrelated strays, so the inheritance idea really didn't fit."

Cotter teamed up with a virologist at Harvard in 1972, and three times that year they went to the woman's home to check on the cats and take blood samples. Cotter was stunned by what they discovered.

"Some of the cats would pick up the virus and later develop leukemia," she said. "Others actually developed antibodies, then became immune, and they never did get the virus or the cancer."

Seven of the cats developed leukemia during the study, providing rather compelling evidence that FeLV was not inherited but rather transmitted.[8] Cotter discovered that the cats who were infected with the virus were immunodeficient. Several of them died of non-cancerous infections.

The knowledge that cats could catch cancer as if it were the common cold revolutionized veterinary care. A test to detect the virus was quickly developed, and used not just by veterinary clinics, but also by animal shelters to separate infected kittens from healthy ones. The first vaccine to treat the virus, developed by an Ohio State University veterinarian, entered the market in the United States in 1985.[9]

Cotter and her colleagues teamed up with pediatric oncologists at the Dana Farber Cancer Institute in Boston to see if there was any evidence that children with leukemia were catching the cancer-causing virus from cats. Thankfully, Cotter said, they didn't find any connection between pediatric and feline leukemia. Still, the legacy of that client and her thirty-five cats lived on, teaching cancer researchers everywhere to consider every eventuality when dealing with this unsolvable disease — and to look to our pets for answers.

"It was the first time anyone found a virus that caused a malignancy in an outbred mammalian species," Cotter said. "Humans are outbred mammalian species. Doing research in inbred mice may be good for studying the mechanism of cancer, but it doesn't apply to humans."

———

Many veterinarians working in the field of comparative oncology believe pets can help them determine the value not just of new drugs, but also of medicines that were not originally intended to treat cancer. They are proponents of drug repurposing — the mission to improve cancer care by using drugs that are already approved and on the market. One of the biggest champions of drug repurposing is Jackie Wypij (pronounced WIH-pee), a veterinarian and professor at the University of Illinois at Urbana-Champaign.

In the spring of 2013, Wypij began recruiting nine cats suffering from cancer for a trial of metformin, a glucose-lowering pill that was first synthesized from a French herb in the 1920s and had been on the market to treat diabetes since 1994.[10] She hoped metformin would prove to be a prime candidate for repurposing as a cancer therapy.

The inspiration for studying metformin's possible utility in oncology was a series of observational studies published in the mid-2000s, which showed that patients with type 2 diabetes who were taking the drug had a lower overall incidence of cancer than people who were not on it. Metformin patients who did develop cancer were less likely to die from the disease than those who didn't take the drug.[11]

No one could say for certain what the connection between metformin and cancer was, though several theories had emerged. Some scientists thought metformin's propensity to improve insulin sensitivity was keeping cancer at bay,[12] while others attributed the effect to the interaction with AMP-activated protein kinase (AMPK), a protein that has been shown in cell cultures to be able to regulate cell metabolism and also to inhibit some tumor development.[13] I wanted to learn more, so I took a trip to Wypij's clinic.

The veterinary school at the University of Illinois is home to nearly five hundred students, and it was clear to me from the moment I walked through the front door of the small animal clinic that learning by doing is the predominant teaching method there. The day I visited the university, the waiting room was filled with several barking dogs, a number of cats in carriers, and two caged parrots whose owners had brought them in for their checkups. Each client was assigned to a fourth-year student, who examined the animal and discussed a potential treatment plan with the veterinarian on duty, who then repeated the exam. (All clients were warned that this process — while instructive for the student — might take a longer than the typical veterinary appointment.)

Whenever a walk-in client arrived, a receptionist would put out a call on the clinic's public address, looking for a student to volunteer for the case.

"Any available orthopedic student, please come to client services," the announcer on the PA system called out, as Wypij and I sat down to talk in a small waiting room just inside the clinic's main entrance. In the background, a dog waiting in an exam room barked impatiently.

The potential value of repurposing metformin for use in veterinary oncology was particularly enticing, Wypij told me. The medicine has a well-established safety profile in people, and, as a generic drug, it is inexpensive, costing just pennies a pill. As most clients pay out-of-pocket for their pets' medical care, veterinarians are eager to not just contribute to the understanding of something that might help people with cancer, but also to expand their own selection of treatments that would be both effective and affordable, she said.

"Drug repurposing is a really great way to use our resources," said Wypij. "Many of the drugs we use are unrelated to cancer but could have anti-cancer effects."

When Wypij first came to the university as an oncology intern in 2004, the school's presence in comparative oncology had been well established by associate professor Timothy M. Fan. He joined the faculty in 1998 and embarked upon several translational research projects, particularly in osteosarcoma. The vet school also had a major presence on the faculty of comparative biosciences, which unites the research efforts of more than a dozen different medical specialists, including epidemiologists, microbiologists, and veterinary surgeons. Together they planned research projects on topics ranging from the use of nanoparticles in drug development to the impact of nutrition and environmental factors on brain development.

Fan supported Wypij's desire to investigate whether old drugs could serve new roles in cancer treatment, he said. But he was realistic about the hurdles she would likely face.

"The challenge is drugs like metformin are what we call chemopreventative — they minimize the likelihood of developing cancer. But that doesn't mean they're necessarily therapeutic," Fan said. "To get those answers, you need to do the experiments."

Wypij decided to test metformin in cats after completing several studies of the drug in tumor samples from both cats and dogs. She discovered that the drug was particularly adept at destroying feline mammary tumor cells and another type of cancer that's similar in cats and humans — oral squamous cell carcinoma (scc). But before she could test the drug in those cancers, she needed to determine the proper dose. So she planned the pilot trial, during which cats with any form of cancer would be given different doses of metformin and then tracked for two weeks.

Even though Wypij needed only nine cats to determine the right dose, she knew finding the right cats would be difficult. That's because all the cats participating in the trial would need to stay in the hospital for up to three days, so Wypij could see how they responded to the drug.

"For some cats it's just not fun to be separated and in a cage where there's dogs barking in the background," Wypij said.

If anyone at the university was up to the challenge of being the cat whisperer, it was Wypij. As a child growing up in Buffalo, New York, Wypij collected Breyer model horses and dreamed of being an equine veterinarian. She didn't become a cat person until she was well into adulthood, but once she jumped into cat ownership, she was hooked, amassing five cats at one point. After she got married and started a family, she let the menagerie of cats dwindle to two.

Wypij sometimes went to heroic lengths for her cats. One day while she was on maternity leave in 2012, Wypij was feeding her infant son when she heard what she thought was her two cats fighting. She went to check out the brawl and discovered that one of the cats, Curly, was choking on a hairball and in a full-blown panic. When Wypij reached in to try to pull the hairball out, Curly bit down so hard he hit a bone in Wypij's hand. Then he went into cardiac arrest.

"I quickly pulled out the hairball from the back of his throat and resuscitated him. Then I put him and the kid in the car and brought them both here," Wypij said, laughing at the memory. After a night on oxygen, Curly survived.

Wypij opened the metformin trial in May 2013 and quickly enrolled Fluffy, a gregarious gray-and-white cat with a type of skin cancer called cutaneous lymphoma.

When I met Fluffy at the university clinic, she was sixteen years old and still undergoing chemotherapy, which had shrunk the once ugly red rash sprawling across most of her chest to a few tiny red bumps. Fluffy's owner, Karol Pichon, kept a small, blue paper collar around the cat's neck at all times, which kept her from licking the affected skin but didn't prevent her from grooming the rest of the thick, luxurious coat that had inspired her name.

When Wypij met Fluffy, she knew immediately the cat would be an ideal candidate for the metformin trial and the hospital stay it required. Fluffy wasn't bothered by loud noises or by being handled by multiple students — a result of having grown up with Pichon's two sons and their rambunctious friends.

"She would be right there in the middle of all of them," Pichon said. "She's always been very friendly. She's not afraid of anybody."

Fluffy was so sociable during the trial the vets and students at the clinic often let her out of her cage so she could roam around. The cat was unflappable, prompting Wypij and her colleagues to nickname her The Fluffinator.

I sat with Pichon in a private client consultation room, and Fluffy ventured out of her cat carrier to explore. She leapt from one leather chair to the other, stopping to balance daintily on the back of the chair where Pichon was sitting. The cat's blue paper collar, known in veterinary circles as an Elizabethan collar, added to her regal stance as she perched on the chair's highest point, lifted her chin, and softly meowed.

Fluffy was still being treated with chemotherapy every

two to three months, and her coat had thinned out a bit as a result, Pichon explained. But the cat was otherwise healthy and living comfortably with her cancer, so Pichon intended to keep her around as long as possible.

Pichon told me she was going through a divorce when she picked Fluffy out from a litter of kittens at a friend's house. The cat saw the family through many more changes, including Pichon losing her accounting job and going back to school to become a hospital medical technician. Fluffy's company was a source of comfort for her, Pichon told me. Saying goodbye would not be easy.

"I'm going to keep doing what I can for her, as long as I'm sure she's not suffering," Pichon said.

At the beginning of the trial, Wypij warned Pichon that the two-week dose of metformin probably wouldn't cure Fluffy's cancer, and it didn't. But entering the cat in the trial was rewarding in other ways, Pichon said. She and the other volunteers each received a credit of $200 to apply to subsequent cancer treatments. The money helped fund Fluffy's chemo.

"I'm a single mom — I didn't have the extra funds to do it," Pichon said. "I was very thankful."

The $200 credit also provided a boost for Robert Nixon and his cat, Stormy, a sixteen-year-old who entered the trial in May 2013 with a cancerous tumor on his ear. Nixon was a retired teacher who spent most of his time volunteering as a humane investigator, helping to bust puppy mills in Illinois and surrounding states. Stormy was one of nine cats and ten dogs living with Nixon on a five-acre home just south of Chicago.

Stormy got his dose of metformin, followed by radiation treatments. The tumor shrank, but eventually returned. Stormy died a few months after the trial, but Nixon never questioned his decision to participate.

"I thought, if it were me I'd do it," Nixon told me when I met him to talk about Stormy.

Nixon originally found Stormy abandoned on a railroad track. One of his legs was mangled and later amputated. The streetwise white-and-gray cat got along on three legs just fine, though he seemed to be happiest sleeping under Nixon's antique Victrola phonograph player.

"If I hadn't had done the trial," Nixon said, "I forever would have wondered if it might have cured the cancer."

Wypij didn't get enough information from that first small trial to be able to speculate whether metformin might be a cure for some cancers. But she hoped to be able to run longer trials to look for signs of the drug's potential as a booster for traditional therapies.

"What if I radiate the cells and then give metformin? Is there an additive or synergistic effect?" she said. "Does it help other forms of chemotherapy kill cancer cells? Or maybe we could use it as a maintenance therapy, to prevent recurrence."

Oncologists on the human side were also intrigued by metformin's potential in cancer. While Wypij was running her trial, a search on ClinicalTrials.gov revealed nearly two hundred studies taking place in the United States and abroad examining whether metformin could be useful in treating colorectal cancer, breast cancer, pancreatic cancer, and several other types.

Wypij hoped that while searching for inexpensive drugs that could be repurposed, she might find an effective therapy for oral squamous cell carcinoma, a highly aggressive and disfiguring tumor that accounts for 10 percent of all cancer diagnoses in cats,[14] and that is virtually identical to head and neck scc, which affects more than forty thousand people in the United States each year.[15] The prognosis in both species is dismal: The five-year survival rate for people diagnosed with head and neck squamous cell carcinoma is 61 percent. The one-year survival rate for cats with the oral form of the disease is just 10 percent.[16]

Because tobacco use is one of the major risk factors for scc in people, veterinarians had long believed cats might provide insight into how smoking causes this tumor type to emerge. That's because cats are like sponges for their environment. Toxins cling to their fur and they ingest them merely by grooming themselves.

One ambitious research project provided strong evidence for the potential value of cats in understanding how the environment affects cancer risk. Using surveys and biopsies from cats diagnosed with oral scc between 1991 and 2000, scientists at Tufts and the University of Massachusetts examined the expression of p53, a gene that normally works to suppress cancer but that commonly becomes mutated in human oral cancers. They found an abnormal accumulation of p53 in cats with oral scc, as well as some association between that genetic overexpression and an exposure to secondhand smoke. This seemed to reinforce studies in people, which reported that both direct and indirect exposure to tobacco correlated with a proliferation of p53 in SCC tumors.[17]

Another study by the same group of researchers revealed an even stronger association between secondhand smoke and feline lymphoma, which is similar to non-Hodgkin's lymphoma in people. Cats who lived in households with smokers had a twofold risk of developing lymphoma. The longer they were exposed to secondhand smoke, the higher their risk. Since studies looking at the impact of tobacco exposure on human lymphoma had been inconclusive, the managers of the cat trial strongly urged the scientific community to take note of their results and to consider further research to clarify the relationship between tobacco and lymphoma.[18]

By the mid-2000s scientists were waking up to the value of feline comparative research and starting more trials. In 2014, for example, clinicians at the University of Tennessee College of Veterinary Medicine in Knoxville teamed up with oncologists at the University of Minnesota in Minneapolis to test a new form of gene therapy to treat SCC. Unlike traditional gene therapy, this treatment wouldn't be delivered by a virus-based vector, nor would it replace a faulty gene with a healthy one. Rather it was a type of RNA designed to interfere with a specific gene called CK2, which churns out a protein that's vital to cell proliferation and survival.[19] CK2 production can go awry in cancer cells, preventing the body from eliminating them.

Because CK2 is essential to both healthy and cancerous cells, targeting it requires a specialized delivery mechanism that can infiltrate cancerous cells yet spare healthy ones. Toward that end, the University of Minnesota researchers designed a nanocapsule that was drawn into the center of cancer cells but that ignored all the healthy cells.

Claire Cannon, assistant professor of oncology at the University of Tennessee's veterinary school, was still recruiting the nine cats she needed for the gene therapy trial when I spoke to her in the summer of 2014, but she was thrilled with the results she had seen in the cats she had treated so far.

"We've seen the disease stabilize in a couple of cats, and we've not seen any significant side effects," she said. "In one patient, the tumor shrank, which was phenomenal."

Cannon's collaborators in Minnesota were in the process of planning a human trial, she told me.

———

At Dartmouth College in Hanover, New Hampshire, a team of microbiologists found a completely different role for cats in the war on cancer. They were creating a cancer therapy from a parasite called Toxoplasma gondii (T. gondii) that's commonly found in cat intestines but rarely causes illness. What T. gondii does do, however, is stimulate the immune system to produce natural killer cells and cytotoxic T cells — both of which destroy cancer cells.

Although cats shed plenty of T. gondii in their feces, it wouldn't be safe to collect the live parasite, grow it, and inject it straight into people, so the Dartmouth team engineered the parasite's DNA. They created a version of it that would act like a cancer vaccine, stimulating the immune system to kill tumor cells without causing any ill effects.

The parasite has some key properties that made this task fairly straightforward. Most importantly, it isn't inherently toxic — its virulence lies mostly in its propensity to replicate inside cells. The Dartmouth team attenuated the parasite so it would grow just enough to stimulate an immune response and would then stop replicating. Then they tested it in mice.

"In mice with intact immune systems, it elicited lifelong immunity after a single vaccination," said David J. Bzik, professor of microbiology and immunology at Dartmouth's Geisel School of Medicine. "It was astonishing."

Bzik's team tested their vaccine in mouse models of melanoma, ovarian cancer, and pancreatic cancer, and each time, it beat back the cancer and produced high rates of survival. When I spoke to Bzik, he and his colleagues were perfecting the vaccine and investigating various methods for improving it. They imagined, for example, being able to personalize it by isolating tumor cells from individual patients and attaching tumor antigens from those cells to the engineered T. gondii parasite. The idea would be to elicit a lifelong immunity in each patient to the particular cancer he or she had.

Bzik, a cat lover with fond memories of two black cats he and his wife once had, could no longer indulge his affection for felines because of his worsening allergies. But he could certainly appreciate the contribution they made to the discovery of what his university dubbed the "cat poop parasite." Once the vaccine was ready for trials, he said, he would start with comparative research in pets.

"It would be a great route to get the human trials going faster," he said.

I figured cats wouldn't be able to participate in those trials because their immune systems would be resistant to T. gondii already, but Bzik told me that wasn't the case. The engineered parasite invades cancer cells so quickly that any antibodies an animal may already have to T. gondii don't have enough time to block it before it performs its job. Therefore the vaccine could very well work in cats with cancer, though he suspected it would prove even more effective in dogs.

To me, it seemed like a prime example of a bunch of creatures that are supposed to be enemies — mice, cats, dogs — unknowingly working together to transform a parasite into a cure for cancer. Bzik agreed with me. And it all started in a litter box.

"Cats," he said, "are truly wonderful creatures."

Chapter 9
A Nose for Detecting Cancer

McBaine is a black-and-white English springer spaniel with a constantly wagging tail and a passion for sniffing out ovarian tumors. During a typical day at the University of Pennsylvania's Vet Working Dog Center in Philadelphia, McBaine is brought into a back room that's mostly bare except for a large metal wheel in the center of the floor. Attached to the wheel are twelve small cups, one of which contains a blood sample from a patient fighting ovarian cancer. McBaine runs around the wheel, smelling each cup one by one, the black tuft on the end of his tail waving happily throughout. Then he stops, places his paw gently on one of the cups, and sits down.

"Good boy!" his trainer yells, as she tosses the dog's favorite rope toy across the floor. Play is McBaine's reward for finding the cancer sample among the cups that contain healthy blood samples or nothing at all.

It was an unusually warm spring day in Philadelphia when I returned to my alma mater to learn about a completely different way dogs are helping in the war on cancer — with their noses. McBaine was one of four dogs enrolled in an innovative study with a lofty goal. After training the dogs to identify ovarian cancer by its smell, the researchers running the project planned to find out exactly what it is the dogs are detecting in the cancer and then invent a diagnostic device that could mimic the dog's nose. That device would give physicians the power to find ovarian cancer long before its victims have any inkling that they are sick.

"We wouldn't put dogs in every hospital or every laboratory," said Cynthia Otto, a veterinarian, dog trainer, and executive director of the Penn Vet Working Dog Center. "Our whole goal is for the end product to be a chemical sensor — a machine with the sensitivity and specificity of the dog."

The Penn Vet Working Dog Center is not on the university's main campus, but two miles away in a nondescript office complex a stone's throw from the Pennsylvania Turnpike. I walked through the main entrance into a giant room with blue foam tiles on the floor and the elements of an obstacle course scattered about — a three-step ladder, a ramp, and several old tires. A dry-erase board on the wall listed all the dogs who were being trained at the center and their progress mastering a variety of skills, from search and rescue, to agility, to impulse control.

As Otto took me on a tour, the sound of the hand-held clickers the dog trainers were using echoed through the halls. The Penn Vet Working Dog Center, she explained, was founded in 2007, but it didn't have its own headquarters until it opened in this building five years later. The center was born from Otto's passion for training search and rescue dogs, which she did in her spare time while working as an emergency veterinarian at Penn. Otto volunteered to provide medical care for the canine search-and-rescue teams that were deployed after Hurricane Floyd hit Florida in 1999, and again in the wake of the September 11th attacks.

After Otto returned from Ground Zero, she got word that the American Kennel Club was looking to fund a study of the 9/11 dogs. She immediately applied, and was chosen to manage the study.

"We've been following the dogs — their health, their behavior. We get x-rays and bloodwork every year, and when the dogs die, we examine the causes of death," Otto said. "As I looked at the whole intersection of dogs and work, I realized there's a lot we don't know."

A decade after 9/11, the Working Dog Center opened its doors with the mission of taking what was learned from the Ground Zero study and others like it to improve the breeding and training of working dogs. The center's trainers started by teaching dogs to detect explosives and narcotics. Later they branched out into the medical realm, pairing dogs who could detect dangerous drops in blood sugar levels with diabetic patients. The cancer-detection project was the center's newest pursuit.

The dogs at Penn's center were named in honor of the dogs and trainers who were deployed to the 9/11 sites, or the victims who died in the act of terrorism. (McBaine's namesake was a search-and-rescue dog who served as part of the control group for the 9/11 canine study.) McBaine and his fellow trainees lived with foster families, who brought them to the center Monday through Friday to be trained.

Otto was a businesslike clinician who, I quickly realized, turned to mush in the presence of her trained dogs. She took me to the back of the center to meet Ffoster, (spelled with a double F), a calm three-year-old yellow Lab who was the newest addition to the cancer-detection program. She was named after 9/11 victim Sandra N. Foster.

"Here's Ffoster, here's the good girl," Otto said, speaking to the dog in a gentle tone as she let her out of the crate where she had been napping. "Do you want to come out and say hi?"

Earlier that day, Ffoster took her turn at the cancer wheel. Ffoster was more deliberate and considerably less bouncy than McBaine, walking slowly around the wheel, checking each cup carefully before coming to a stop. She was right. She got a treat as a reward.

"You did good today," Otto cooed. "You're learning good stuff."

The notion that dogs might be able to detect cancer first emerged in 1989, when the prestigious British medical journal *The Lancet* published a five-paragraph letter titled "Sniffer dogs in the melanoma clinic?" In the letter, two physicians at King's College Hospital in London described the case of a forty-four-year-old woman, who came into their clinic with a lesion on her left thigh. She told them she made the appointment because her dog, a Doberman–border collie mix, was constantly sniffing a mole on her leg.[1]

The dog, the physicians wrote, "showed no interest in the other moles on the patient's body but frequently spent several minutes a day sniffing intently at the lesion, even through the patient's trousers."

One day the woman donned shorts, at which point her dog tried to bite the mole off completely. That's when she decided she should get it examined. The object of the dog's obsession turned out to be a malignant melanoma.

"Perhaps malignant tumours such as melanoma, with their aberrant protein synthesis, emit unique odours which, though undetectable to man, are easily detected by dogs," the physicians wrote.

They reported that the dog had saved the patient's life, because when she came into the clinic the tumor was so small they could easily treat it. She was cured.

Those five paragraphs were enough to mobilize dog-loving scientists all over the world to design studies testing whether dogs can smell cancer. Over the next several years, dozens of papers were published in medical journals, most of them reporting astounding success rates — often with 90 percent accuracy or better — among dogs trained to sniff cancer.

Otto read those papers avidly and watched with fascination as other dog-training organizations began teaching dogs to sniff cancer. She wanted to do the same, she just didn't have the funding or the know-how she needed to get started.

Then one day shortly after the new center opened, Otto's phone rang. It was a cold call from another Penn faculty member, ophthalmologist Jody R. Piltz-Seymour, a dog lover who had also been captivated by all the reports about dogs who could sniff cancer. Piltz-Seymour had lost her father and aunt to pancreatic cancer. A second aunt and her mother-in-law both died of ovarian cancer.

Piltz-Seymour was particularly interested in research done by a Swedish scientist named György Horvath. In a 2008 paper, Horvath described how he trained a four-year-old black giant schnauzer to recognize tissue samples from late-stage ovarian cancer patients by their scent. Then Horvath ran the dog through two series of tests to see if she could tell the difference between ovarian cancer and healthy tissue, even when the cancer samples were taken from women in the early stages of the disease. In both testing situations, the dog correctly identified all the cancerous samples, and when presented with 80 pieces of healthy tissue, only twice did she falsely identify them as cancerous.[2]

Horvath's results made Piltz-Seymour realize dogs could be the key to early detection, but she knew she would need help translating the findings into a useful clinical tool. Then the Working Dog Center opened, and she figured she had nothing to lose by giving it a shot.

"I thought we had this phenomenal new resource right in the backyard," Piltz-Seymour said. As she reminisced about her cold call to Otto, she began to laugh. "You have to picture this — here's an ophthalmologist calling about dogs and cancer."

Little did she know that Otto was already keen on the idea and was looking for an ally to help get a study started.

"Jody had done a lot of research and wanted to see if she could help move it forward," Otto said. "She spearheaded this — it was personal."

Piltz wanted to start with ovarian cancer, not just because of her family history, but also because she believed it was where the dogs could make the most impact.

"Everybody in my family succumbed to their cancers because none of their cancers were caught early," Piltz-Seymour told me. "The vast majority of the time, ovarian cancer is caught late. But when caught early, the success rate with treatment is brilliant. That makes it the perfect cancer to study."

Indeed, the five-year survival rate for ovarian cancer patients who are diagnosed and treated before their cancer spreads is 92 percent. Yet only 15 percent of ovarian cancers are found that early.[3] These tumors rarely produce symptoms in their early stages, and when they do, their victims commonly mistake what they're feeling for something far more benign, like constipation.

As I listened to Piltz-Seymour talk about this conundrum, I thought about Beth, who didn't know she was gravely ill until her cancer had spread beyond her stomach.

"Gastric cancer is similar to ovarian cancer in that it doesn't produce symptoms until it's too late," I told Piltz-Seymour.

The five-year survival rate for gastric cancer patients who are diagnosed at the earliest stages is as high as 71 percent.[4] That's because surgery and chemo can be quite effective when the cancer hasn't spread. The problem is, the only good way to find stomach tumors is with an endoscopy, an invasive and sometimes risky procedure that involves sticking a tiny camera down the patient's throat while he or she is sedated.

In most countries, healthy people aren't given an endoscopy unless they have a strong family history of gastric cancer. Because we had no history of the disease in our family, the doctors who saw Beth for her checkups and minor complaints never would have imagined they should look in her stomach for signs of trouble. So they didn't.

In Japan, where the prevalence of gastric cancer is high, mass screening is routine, and now half of all cases of the disease are found in the early stages. Hence the five-year survival rate following surgery for Japanese patients is a staggering 96 to 99 percent.[5]

Whenever I see dogs like McBaine sticking their noses into human tissue samples and instantly identifying the cancerous ones or I read about them in the press, I have a fantasy: I imagine everyone in the world going to the doctor for a routine physical each year and breathing into a tube, or leaving a blood or urine sample, and learning on the spot if there's any sign of cancer in their stomachs, lungs, ovaries, or anywhere else in the body where tumors can easily hide. If dogs can detect cancer, then it seems only logical that scientists can unlock the mysteries of the canine sense of smell and replicate it with a diagnostic device — an electronic nose that could be put to work in every medical clinic in the world, but that wouldn't need to be fed and walked twice a day.

Piltz-Seymour told me she had exactly the same fantasy.

"I kept seeing these very interesting articles about dogs detecting cancer, but no one seemed to follow through to develop anything that could be used in clinical practice," she said.

When she set out to develop an early-detection system for ovarian cancer, Piltz-Seymour knew she needed to put together a team that included more than just dog trainers. She began calling and e-mailing oncologists and doctors, most of whom ignored her. Then she got a return call from a gynecologist at Penn named Janos L. Tanyi. He offered to join the team and referred Piltz-Seymour to two other Penn faculty members he believed would be interested: molecular scientist George Preti and physics professor A.T. Charlie Johnson. Preti and Johnson had already done some research to try to identify the odors associated with ovarian cancer. They both jumped at the opportunity to add dogs to their team.

"Our initial hypothesis that ovarian cancer would emanate a unique odor signature was based on the work done in Europe with dogs," said Preti, who in addition to his appointment at Penn was a scientist at the Monell Chemical Senses Center, a Philadelphia research house devoted entirely to unlocking the mysteries of smell and taste. "I knew dogs would be a very good biological detector."

———

The dog's nose is among the most powerful sensory organs the world has ever known. Dogs have 200 million olfactory receptors (ORs), which are proteins on the surface of the neurons inside their noses that help their brains to perceive and process odors.[6] Humans, by contrast, have just five million ORs. The mucous membranes inside dogs' nostrils are extraordinarily dense, and their noses exquisitely structured for the efficient processing of smells. That allows them to detect odors that are present in quantities as low as parts per trillion — an amount so minuscule it's almost impossible to imagine. On top of that, many experts believe the proportion of the dog's brain that's dedicated to analyzing scents is 40 times larger than that of humans.[7] Suffice it to say, it's enough for scientists to estimate that the dog's ability to recognize minute traces of particular odors is one million times better than that of people.[8]

But what exactly are the dogs sniffing in cancer that they find so alarming? Shortly after *The Lancet* publication, a popular theory emerged suggesting that tumors must be emitting volatile organic compounds (VOCs), which are carbon-based chemicals that naturally occur in the body. Since the late 1980s, scientists have identified a variety of VOCs that are overly abundant in cancerous tissues, including some types of benzene.[9]

Because VOCs have a low boiling point, they easily evaporate and travel to places far from the original tumor, including through urine, blood, and exhaled breath.[10] As the scientific world became aware of the dog's ability to sniff cancer, some researchers set out to prove that tumors have unique VOC signatures, or specific odor profiles that distinguish them from healthy tissue and that can be easily detected and analyzed — if not by dogs than by some sort of non-invasive test.

Among those researchers were scientists at the Cleveland Clinic, who in the early 2000s collected breath samples from lung cancer patients, healthy volunteers, and patients with other lung diseases. They analyzed the exact chemical makeup of the cancerous breath and used it to develop a device containing thirty-two tiny sensors.

There are two criteria used to judge the value of a diagnostic test in oncology: sensitivity and specificity. A sensitive test can pick up the presence of cancer. A specific test can do so with a high rate of accuracy — meaning it rarely detects the disease in people who don't have it.[11]

Back when the Cleveland Clinic was doing its study, PET scanning in lung cancer was 97 percent specific and 78 percent sensitive.[12] The Cleveland Clinic's electronic nose stacked up pretty well, scoring 92 percent specificity and 71 percent sensitivity. That means the electronic nose missed the abnormality about a third of the time, but when it found something fishy, it was nearly flawless at figuring out when it was cancer and when it was not.[13]

The dogs also performed well. In a 2012 trial of breath samples from 220 people, sniffer dogs scored 90 percent on sensitivity and 72 percent on specificity for lung cancer, even when the scientists tried to confuse them with samples from patients with the non-cancerous lung condition known as chronic obstructive pulmonary disorder (COPD). Other dog studies that had trained dogs with urine, blood, or tissue samples achieved comparable or better results in detecting melanoma, as well as ovarian, breast, bladder, and colorectal cancer. [14]

As it became more and more clear that dogs could smell cancer, some researchers wondered if it really made sense to spend time and money creating electronic noses. Some thought a smarter strategy would be to employ the dogs themselves in medical clinics as a sort of living warning system — an advance guard to alert doctors and patients that further testing would be a good idea.

One such researcher was Robert Gordon, an obstetrician and gynecologist at Scripps Health in La Jolla, California. Gordon envisioned equipping volunteer church groups, for example, with urine-collection kits and a few dogs who were trained to sniff them.

"If anybody came up positive then they could be sent to a center where they could get more sophisticated testing," he said. "I thought in areas that were not developed, in the backwoods, you could use a dog."

Gordon, who is hearing impaired, was inspired by his own dog, a Chihuahua-beagle mix named Ginger, whom he had trained to be a certified hearing-assistance dog.

"She's a fabulous animal," Gordon said. "She goes everywhere with me — restaurants, movies — helping me as a hearing dog. I put a towel down so her hair doesn't get on anything. She snores through the loud movies."

In 2004, Gordon set out to train Ginger and nine other dogs to discriminate between patients who had prostate cancer, those who had breast cancer, and those who were healthy, based on urine samples. The dogs made a lively crew that included a miniature goldendoodle, an Italian greyhound, and a Pembroke Welsh corgi. But few of them showed much talent for sniffing cancer — only two performed better than chance, or luck, at specificity in detecting each of the two tumor types. None were better than chance at sensitivity, not even Ginger.[15]

After thinking about it, Gordon concluded that the

imperfections were not in the dogs themselves but rather in the way he had designed the study. He could only gather a few urine samples, which he froze, thawed, and re-used several times during the training process. He wondered if all that freezing and thawing might have destroyed the scents he was training the dogs to recognize. He had also discovered that the dogs would get fatigued after less than two hours of work. It all made Gordon realize that developing an electronic nose might indeed be far wiser than using dogs at medical clinics or in the backwoods.

"It's impractical to spend the money on dogs," Gordon said. "That money would be best served finding what the chemicals are that the cancer puts off — the chemical signature that makes them so destructive."

Other researchers had already discovered that finding the VOCs was the easy part. The hard part was figuring out how to train a machine to recognize cancer VOCs amid the thousands of other scents emitted by the human body. In dogs, that process is known as imprinting, and it involves teaching the animals to recognize the scent of cancer simply by exposing them to it. Much like a bloodhound who's directed to find a missing child might be presented with a t-shirt infused with that child's scent, a cancer-detection dog is asked to sniff cancerous tissue, or samples of urine, blood or breath from sick patients, and then taught to find that scent while ignoring everything else.

As the research papers proving the dog's ability to sniff cancer continued to pile up, a handful of scientists took on the challenge of developing an electronic nose that could be imprinted with the scent of cancer as effectively as a dog's could. Among the most passionate scientists in that pursuit was someone in my sister's backyard: Hossam Haick, a professor at the Technion-Israel Institute of Technology in Haifa, Israel.

In 2007, Haick began developing a device he dubbed Na-Nose, short for nanotechnology nose. He used tiny gold particles to create an array of electronic sensors, which were connected to a tube. The result was a device that operated much like a breathalyzer, but was far more sensitive because it could analyze up to one thousand different gases in exhaled breath. Haick set out to prove that the Na-Nose could detect much more than the mere presence of cancer — that it could also distinguish one form of the disease from another.

Haick's main challenge, he told me, was figuring out how to deal with all the confounding molecules, as he called them, that appear in breath, like mouthwash ingredients, or residual odors from the garlic pizza a patient ate two days before taking the breath test (and failed to eliminate with the mouthwash). Haick, a chemical engineer, used artificial intelligence to train the Na-Nose to recognize cancer VOCs and ignore everything else. Over the next few years, Haick and his colleagues tested their device in clinics around the world, recruiting four thousand patients with a variety of different cancers to try it.

The results were often remarkable. For instance, in 2012, Haick teamed up with scientists in China and Latvia to test his technology in 130 patients with stomach disorders. Thirty-seven of the patients had gastric cancer, while the rest had ulcers or a benign condition. They found that the

Na-Nose technology could distinguish between the cancerous and non-cancerous diseases with 83 percent sensitivity and 96 percent specificity. Even better, it could pick out the patients who had early-stage gastric cancer from those who were in the late stages of the disease with 89 percent sensitivity and 94 percent specificity. The Na-Nose's accuracy was consistent regardless of the patients' tobacco and alcohol consumption — habits that had the potential to produce confounding odors.[16]

I told Haick about my sister and asked if he thought his device might someday be used to screen healthy people, allowing stomach tumors to be detected even when they're completely silent.

"Absolutely," he replied. "That is our intention. We want to catch the cancer at the early stages before anybody has symptoms. Then we can increase the survival rate by using currently available treatments. It's true with other cancers, too."

In a later study, presented at a medical meeting on stomach disorders in the summer of 2014, the Na-Nose performed even better, distinguishing gastric cancer from ulcers and pre-cancerous lesions with 98 percent specificity.[17]

Haick's technology proved equally adept at discerning lung cancer, often performing better than sniffer dogs or the Cleveland Clinic's early rendition of an electronic nose. In a study published in 2012, for example, the Na-Nose could determine whether the nodules found in patients with lung disorders were benign or cancerous with 86 percent sensitivity and 96 percent specificity.[18]

"If you detect the lung cancer at the early stages you can increase the survival rate from 10 percent to more than 70 percent," Haick said. "But only by early detection."

Cure rates improve even more when lung tumors possess genetic mutations that can be addressed with targeted therapies. So Haick set out to prove his nanosensors could detect the abnormal VOC patterns associated with those mutations. In 2013, his group published a paper describing what they called the volatile fingerprints of three well-known lung cancer mutations — KRAS, EGFR, and EML4-ELK. By this time, there were already drugs on the market that improved survival times for patients with those mutations.[19]

One day in late 2012, Haick's phone rang. On the other end of the line was Steve Lerner, a Boston-based entrepreneur and veteran of the semiconductor industry. Lerner had kept coming across Haick's research in the scientific literature on nanotechnology and was convinced he could commercialize the Na-Nose technology through his start-up, Alpha Szenszor, which had patented a different nanotech-based system to detect VOCs in breath. Lerner was particularly interested in developing a breath test to detect lung cancer. Within two months, he and Haick had formed a joint venture.

When I caught up with Lerner in the summer of 2014, he was working on expanding the joint venture with Haick and the Technion-Israel Institute to include a sensor for gastric cancer. He told me he was particularly impressed with the data on gastric cancer coming out of Haick's lab. And he had big plans for the product he wanted to develop.

"Anybody should be able to walk into a drug store and for twenty-five bucks get a lung cancer or a gastric cancer screen that gives them a 90 percent accuracy," Lerner said. "And it should be part of an annual physical. Ten minutes of breathing into a tube — it's that simple."

Perhaps, but turning the dream into reality wasn't that simple for Lerner's company. He believed he could build a device, test it in a few hundred patients, and get FDA approval within eighteen months. But he had to put the project on hold after being repeatedly turned down by investors. The problem, Lerner said, was that the Na-Nose was such a new and untested idea, investors thought it too risky a gamble. Lerner had the door slammed in his face by so many American investors, he said, that he was starting to approach investors in Asia and Europe instead.

Lerner was inspired by his personal experience with cancer, which included losing his forty-year-old brother to colon cancer. Then his mother was diagnosed with a brain tumor.

"Both of these could have been caught in much earlier states with the type of diagnostic we are working on," he said.

That's why Lerner was undeterred by all the rejection from investors.

"I'm looking at this as a point of pride. I will see it through," he said.

Two women — seventeen hundred miles and worlds apart from each other — were not willing to wait for the medical industry to turn the power of the dog's nose into an approved medical device. They were both dog trainers who had experienced cancer up close, and, unknown to each other, they were steadfastly pursuing separate ideas for using sniffer dogs in the war on cancer. At first, I admit, I pegged them as dreamers. I tended to agree with Gordon and other scientists who had told me it was not feasible to put dogs to work in any medical setting. But as I got to know these women, and I thought about how different Beth's fate might have been if her cancer had been caught early, I wondered if maybe they were on to something big.

The first was Donna Waugh, president of the American Scent Dog Association (ASDA) in Little Rock, Arkansas. When I spoke with her in the summer of 2014, she was developing a plan to train dogs to recognize the scent of various cancers, and then deploy them as service dogs for survivors of the disease. She already had one interested survivor: a woman working in Washington, D.C., in a high-profile government position, who had contacted ASDA looking for peace of mind after surviving thyroid cancer.

"She's in remission, but she told me the cancer had taken away her confidence," Waugh said.

A service dog trained to detect cancer could routinely sniff her urine samples, and then reassure her that every headache or fever or twinge of discomfort she felt wasn't the cancer coming back, Waugh said.

"From a simple urine test she could do at home, the dog can tell her, 'You're fine, don't worry, you're fine.'"

Waugh, who started her dog-training career working in search and rescue, learned about the potential of dogs in medical settings the hard way in 2006. One afternoon she came home from work with a blinding headache. She went to lie down on the couch, but her border collie, Harrison, refused to let her rest.

"I just wanted to go to sleep. I could hardly see straight," Waugh said. "Harrison was like, 'You won't lie down.'"

Fearing the dog might be telling her that the headache was a sign of something serious, Waugh checked herself in to the local hospital.

"My dog sent me here," she told the nurse. "I think I'm going to die."

Doctors quickly discovered that Waugh had blood clots in her brain that could have been fatal had she lain down on the couch and fallen asleep instead of checking herself in. She was put on a blood thinner, and she survived.

During that medical ordeal, one of Waugh's physicians became concerned about a benign tumor on her uterus that a scan revealed. The doctor wanted to remove the tumor to make sure it hadn't turned cancerous. But Waugh told him that the tumor had been discovered years earlier and she knew she it wasn't cancerous because Harrison hadn't alerted her that anything was wrong. By 2011, however, the tumor had grown to ten pounds and was pressing on her ovaries, so she agreed to the operation.

"It was a nightmare, and a risky surgery," Waugh said. "But the dog was right. I did not have cancer."

Shortly thereafter, Waugh teamed up with doctors at the University of Arkansas for Medical Sciences to train her second border collie, John D, to detect ovarian cancer. Later they expanded their research to include more dogs, and trained them to detect thyroid cancer, as well. The dogs' accuracy matched that of dogs trained by other research groups around the world, Waugh said.

Waugh set out to prove that there should be a new type of medical service dog — one who could prevent cancer recurrences from turning deadly. Her plan was to imprint dogs with the scents of different tumors and teach them words that their new owners could use to command them to go to work.

For fellow dog trainer Dina Zaphiris, the motivation to make something great out of dogs' amazingly good sense of smell came from her mother, who fought and lived with breast cancer for twenty years before succumbing to the disease in 2010. Zaphiris, the founder of the In Situ Foundation in Malibu, California, trained dogs to detect breast, lung, and ovarian cancer in both breath and blood samples. Her goal was to develop a breath test that women could do at home and then send to a central location to be analyzed by a team of dogs.

Zaphiris wasn't opposed to the idea of developing an automated device — in fact, she was one of the first dog trainers hired by a scientist who wanted to do just that. In 2003, the Pine Street Foundation in San Anselmo, California, recruited her and another dog trainer to help design a trial that involved training dogs to sniff lung and breast tumors at various stages. The trial showed that the dogs could detect lung cancer with 99 percent specificity and sensitivity and breast cancer with 88 percent sensitivity and 98 percent specificity. The dogs were accurate at all four stages of cancer, and using Zaphiris's methods, they could be easily trained in a matter of weeks.[20]

Zaphiris was impressed but impatient. She didn't want to wait for someone to figure out how to transform Pine Street's findings into a diagnostic tool.

"If they can develop a machine that's sensitive and specific, bravo. I'll be the first in line to get screened," she told me. "But until we have a machine that can do that before the cancer is in stage four, people who want to have screenings done by the dogs should be able to have that done. The only thing that's important to me right now is that the dogs can do it — and they can do it better than any machine."

The device that Zaphiris envisioned was a tube that would collect a breath sample and transfer it to a cloth, which would be sent by overnight mail to her training facility. A team of dogs would sniff it, give their verdict, and the customer would have an answer the next day.

Zaphiris was preparing to apply for FDA clearance to develop her product when I spoke to her. She knew she was facing huge challenges. The history of at-home medical tests was rife with obstacles. Consider the common pregnancy test, for example. The tools to make it a reality were developed in the late 1960s, but the first at-home test wasn't cleared for marketing until 1977.[21] A simple at-home saliva test for HIV was first proposed in 1994[22] but was so controversial the first such test kit didn't make it to the market until 2012.[23]

Perhaps the biggest warning to anyone hoping to commercialize a diagnostic test for sniffing out cancer — whether it's done by a machine or the dogs themselves — came in late 2013, when the FDA sent a stern warning letter to 23andMe, a California company that had been marketing an at-home genome mapping kit. The product used saliva samples from customers to forecast, based on their genes, their risk of developing 254 diseases, including heart disease, diabetes, and breast cancer. The FDA chastised the company for failing to properly validate its testing methods and expressed concerns about how customers who received false information would react. The agency demanded that 23andMe pull its test from the market immediately, which it did.[24]

Zaphiris conceded that she may never achieve FDA approval for her cancer test, but she had to keep trying. As word got out about what her foundation was planning, her e-mail inbox filled up with pleas from women who wanted the dogs to sniff their breath samples. Many had lesions show up on their mammograms that were too tiny to be examined any further, she said.

"They're told they have to sit at home and wait for four months to see if those pods grow into tumors, because they're too small to biopsy," Zaphiris said.

"In cases like that, the dogs would be extremely valuable in helping to at least ease somebody's mind."

Zaphiris had to turn down all those requests. The liability risk was too high, she said, and managing the potential for lawsuits was something she needed to figure out how to do. After all, what would happen if one of the dogs were wrong?

"Nothing is 100 percent," she said. "There will still be the 1 percent that we miss or give a false positive. But we could have [customers] sign a waiver. It should be up to each individual person to decide what they want to do with the results."

Despite her family history of breast cancer, Zaphiris told me she had no reason to believe she faced a higher risk than the average woman of developing the disease. Still, she was concerned that she would not be adequately protected by her regular mammograms.

"Mammograms miss. My mom's mammogram missed her cancer all together — she found the lump herself," Zaphiris said. "I try not to worry about it, but yeah, I'm scared every day, because I've seen it happen. If it were up to me, I would get my breasts checked by these dogs."

———

In 2009, Claire Guest's five-year-old yellow Labrador retriever, Daisy, suddenly started behaving oddly. When Guest opened up the back door of her car to let the dog out for a run at a park near their home in Buckinghamshire, England, Daisy jumped at her. Guest batted the Lab away, but Daisy kept on slamming into Guest's chest, over and over again.

Guest, a psychologist and dog trainer who started her career by training dogs to assist the hearing impaired, knew better than to ignore Daisy's strange behavior. A few years earlier, Guest had contributed to a research project that trained six dogs to recognize bladder cancer in urine samples.[25] She went on to train dozens more dogs, including Daisy, who became a master at detecting bladder, prostate, and kidney tumors. Guest became CEO of Medical Detection Dogs, a charitable organization that trained dogs to recognize signs of cancer and a host of other diseases, including diabetes.

"I had to keep pushing Daisy away," Guest said. "As I did that I felt a sore patch in my breast, like a bruise really. I felt it for the next few days, and it wasn't going away."

Guest had not yet had her first mammogram when she found the lump that Daisy had been trying to tell her she had. A biopsy came back negative, but further tests indicated it might be cancerous. Guest had the lump removed, and she underwent radiation therapy.

"I was diagnosed with a very deep breast cancer," Guest said. "It probably would have taken a couple of years for me to feel it. Had Daisy not drawn my attention to it, things would have been very different."

Over the ensuing years, Guest and her colleagues completed several more studies, training hundreds of dogs to detect a wide variety of cancers, and advising other researchers who were trying to build electronic noses, including Haick. Guest's priority, she told me, was to prove that the dog's cancer-sniffing ability was durable, meaning it could be counted on time after time to be both sensitive and specific, and that there would be no question that the dog was detecting the disease and nothing else.

"The problem some groups have is that if you look at the numbers of samples that the dogs have screened, it's small," Guest said. "What happens is they learn a person and they latch onto that scent. If you ask a dog to screen the same sample twenty times, the first time, he's probably making a true detection. But after that, he'll just be remembering that person."

Over the course of five years, Guest tested Daisy's cancer-detection ability on six thousand different samples, keeping meticulous records on exactly what happened each time the dog sniffed the tissue samples at the headquarters of Medical Detection Dogs. Daisy, sleek and graceful as she walked down a line of samples placed in small buckets on the floor, paused whenever she thought she smelled the cancer, bowing her head to sniff once, then again to confirm, and sitting down for the treat that would tell her she was right.

"Daisy's sensitivity and specificity was over 90 percent," Guest said. "So we're starting to see what the dog's real ability is."

Guest's own cancer scare encouraged her to press on with her work.

"It inspired me to keep going at a time when this idea wasn't easily accepted," she said. "I made it my mission to train my dogs to do this work."

Not long after Guest completed her cancer treatment, she told her story at a conference on working dogs in Belgium. In the audience that day was Cindy Otto, who was mesmerized by Guest's story. The University of Pennsylvania had yet to open its dog-training facility, but Otto knew even back then that combating cancer through early detection would be part of her mission.

"As I listened to Claire Guest, I started thinking about

what the possibilities were for these dogs," Otto said. "That's what planted the seeds."

From the very first meeting Otto had with Piltz-Seymour and the rest of her founding team, it was clear they would need to plan several stages of research in order to complete the full circuit — from proving the dogs could detect ovarian cancer to developing the device that would mimic that ability.

Otto told me the plan was first to train the dogs to recognize ovarian cancer with a high degree of sensitivity and specificity. Then, using Preti's and Johnson's discoveries about the vocs that seem to be prevalent in ovarian tumors, Otto would present those chemicals, one by one, to the dogs, to see if they could discern the exact compounds that produce the cancer's unique scent.

"If there is some way we can identify that, then we can facilitate the generation of an effective sensor," she said.

Otto was amazed by how fast her dogs were learning to detect cancer. As we sat in her small office next to the blue-tiled training room, she pulled up a video of Tsunami, a lumbering German shepherd who so far was more accurate than any of her other dogs at detecting ovarian cancer. I could not meet Tsunami that day — she was a dog who preferred working over socializing with strangers, Otto told me apologetically — but it was clear from the video that this dog had mastered her job.

Tsunami walked slowly from one cup to the next, stopping after just a few and sitting down decisively, without even checking the other samples to be sure she had found the right one. She was rewarded with her favorite rope toy.

"She's not going to check them all and then go back," Otto said. "She'll stop wherever the cancer is."

Completing all the planned stages of the research would be a Herculean task — and one that the Penn team did not have adequate funding to complete. When they first formulated their plan, Piltz-Seymour started writing grant applications and sending them to every ovarian cancer charity she could find. She scored an early victory with the award of an $80,000 grant from the Kaleidoscope of Hope Ovarian Cancer Foundation. The team used the money to generate their first round of data. When I spoke to Piltz-Seymour in the summer of 2014, she was struggling to raise more funding.

"I would love to find a generous donor who has a love of dogs and believes in the potential they can bring to fighting cancer," she told me.

She admitted that after having lost so many of her family members to the disease, she was torn between the two approaches: the practicality of an automated nose, which would take many years to develop and bring to market, and just using the dogs themselves to detect cancer.

"We are all about creating the technology," she said. "But if the dogs can do it now with the proper training, why not harness their abilities now?"

Chapter 10
Countless Canines, One Health

The battle cry to enlist dogs in cancer research is being heard around the world — a trend I recognized with the very first dog whose story I uncovered: Basil the golden retriever. Basil's owners, Alan and Kathy Wilber, had told me about UC Davis veterinarian Gillian Dank, an Israeli who was completing her education in the United States, and whose gentle guidance through their dog's amputation and cancer treatments brought them great comfort. Dank was an oncology resident from 2000 to 2002, during which time she worked with Cheryl London on the Palladia trials and other comparative studies. Then she returned to Israel to work as a full-time veterinary oncologist.

I had spent the better part of a year meeting the scientists and dog owners who were involved in comparative oncology research when I started planning a vacation to Israel — my first trip back since my sister died three years earlier. It would be a family vacation with my parents and my then-fiancé, Harry, who would be meeting the Israeli side of my family for the first time.

I knew Dank had done some comparative oncology trials of her own since she returned to Israel — I had found papers about her work in medical journals — and I was curious to learn more about her experiences. So just before we left, I contacted Dank and invited her to join me for coffee one day during my visit.

Dank lived down the street from where we were staying in Beth's family's home in Tel Aviv, and she readily agreed to meet me. We met at a bright outdoor café, where the benches were adorned with carvings of dogs at play. I'm not a believer in divine intervention, but I couldn't help but wonder if my sister sent me to this particular café to meet this particular veterinarian, so I could see that even in the tiny country of Israel, dogs were being enlisted in the war on cancer.

Dank was born in Connecticut and moved with her family to Israel at the age of 14, she told me. She earned her undergraduate and veterinary degrees at Hebrew University and realized in her last year of schooling that she wanted to help pets with cancer. At the time, there wasn't a single veterinarian in Israel who specialized in oncology. So she applied for the UC Davis residency with the intention of learning all that she could from some of the world's top cancer specialists, then using that know-how to improve the outlook for dogs and cats with cancer in her home country. Dank hadn't had much exposure to comparative oncology until she landed at Davis.

Dank told me that Basil had been a big inspiration to her, because before he entered the trial, it wasn't clear to her, London, or anyone else on the research team that the experimental drug would be of any value at all.

"We were passing any dog that we thought was appropriate over to Cheryl London for the trial, and not very many of them responded to the drug," Dank said. "Basil's response was amazing. I realized that comparative oncology wasn't just about dogs being better models than lab rats — it was also about helping the dogs. I thought that was wonderful."

Israel is a nation of just eight million people and 387,000 dogs.[1] It is dwarfed by the United States, home to 314 million people and a remarkably huge canine population of eighty-three million.[2] So I was not surprised when Dank told me she was proud of what she had been able to achieve in comparative oncology so far.

"I've only been back ten years, and we've already run five different trials," Dank said. "That's not too bad."

Just as Dank's career was taking off, medical professionals around the world were starting to embrace the idea that improving animal health could have broad beneficial effects on human health. Comparative oncology is part of this movement, known as the One Health Initiative. The goal of One Health is to bring together professionals from all medical disciplines and to promote the sharing of knowledge and advances related to all the illnesses that animals and people share, from infectious diseases to cancer.

Veterinarian Calvin W. Schwabe was among the first to champion the idea of One Health, which he first proposed in 1964 and then featured in his textbook *Veterinary Medicine and Human Health*. Schwabe directed the World

Health Organization's (WHO) research programs on parasitic diseases and served as the founding chair of UC Davis's department of epidemiology and preventive medicine. But it wasn't until the 2000s that WHO and other organizations began to aggressively encourage veterinarians and doctors to work together. In 2007, One Health got a major boost when the American Medical Association passed a resolution promoting partnerships between veterinarians and doctors who treat people.[3]

Israel was an early and enthusiastic supporter of One Health. In 2006, for example, Israeli physicians and veterinarians collaborated with their counterparts in Jordan and the Palestinian territories to contain an outbreak of avian flu on commercial poultry farms. In a journal article, a veterinarian from Hebrew University and two physicians specializing in pubic health recounted the avian flu collaboration as one example of how cross-discipline (and in that case, cross-border) partnerships validate the One Health approach. One Health, they wrote, "is extremely important in a variety of fields, including enhancement of breakthroughs in biomedical research, epidemiological studies and public health policy decision-making. Combining different skills and ways of thinking acquired in the two disciplines can lead to a synergistic process of brainstorming and very valuable exchanges of ideas."[4]

It was in this welcoming environment that Dank began planning comparative oncology trials. One of her first collaborations was with a company called InSightec, which had developed a surgical technology that used magnetic resonance–guided, high-intensity ultrasound beams to vaporize tumors and other diseased tissue. Dank worked with the company to try the technology in several dogs, including a 10-year-old mixed-breed dog with a liver tumor. They demonstrated that the device shrank some areas of the tumor, and in a later journal article about the case they suggested potential improvements to the technique.[5] InSightec went on gain several regulatory approvals for its ultrasound technology, including U.S. and European licenses for its use in treating patients whose cancer had spread to their bones.

Dank told me she occasionally turned down requests from other companies that wanted to test unproven cancer treatments in dogs. Like so many of the veterinarians I had met in the United States, she wanted to make it clear that comparative oncology is only ethical when dogs with cancer stand to benefit as much as human patients do.

"It's not just about doing what's good for science or for people," she said. "What about the actual dogs who are going to be in the study? We don't want to do anything unless it's in their best interest."

A few years after the InSightec trial, Dank got an offer to do a comparative study for Efranat, a local biotech start-up founded by Avi Levin and Boaz Shoham. Both had lost their wives to cancer, and they were determined to improve the outlook for future cancer patients. So they launched the company in 2009, named it for their wives, Anat and Efrat, and began looking for an experimental drug to develop.

When I heard Levin and Shoham's story, I immediately felt a kinship with them. They were not scientists — Levin was a pilot and Shoham an architect — but they were so driven by their personal losses that they took time off from their careers to venture into biotechnology, hungry for the opportunity to contribute to cancer research. After Beth died, I quit one steady journalism job with benefits, then a second, so I could take the time I needed to learn the story of comparative oncology and bring attention to it by writing this book. I had not met these men, but I understood their need to step out of their grief and turn their losses into something positive.

When Dank first learned about Efranat's drug, she was skeptical, she told me. A scientist in Philadelphia, Nobuto Yamamoto, had developed the drug, but he was boasting that it could be a cure for all cancers. The drug was a protein called GcMAF — a little-known molecule that Dank doubted could be the magic bullet that Yamamoto claimed it was.

Yamamoto had published papers on three small trials of the drug in people with cancer.[6] There were so few patients in those trials that no firm conclusions could be drawn about whether GcMAF actually worked. But Dank was willing to test it in dogs with cancer, especially since she could tell from those initial studies in people that the drug hadn't caused any dangerous side effects.

"We have so many cases that come in and are hopeless. It didn't hurt to try it," she said.

Of the fourteen dogs Dank treated with the experimental drug, nine responded positively to it. Two of those dogs Dank would never forget, she told me.

The first was an Irish setter who came to Dank's clinic

covered in ugly red rings — the hallmark of the skin cancer cutaneous lymphoma.

"It's the kind of disease where they're supposed to be dead within four months," she said.

She treated the Irish setter with GcMAF and the red rings disappeared. Three years after the experimental treatment, the dog was alive and still cancer-free.

"Another dog came in that I shouldn't have put on the study. He was about to die," Dank said.

That dog had metastatic squamous-cell carcinoma. Even though the disease is not as common in dogs as it is in cats and people, it's yet another cancer that, in its latter stages, is incurable.

"His entire stomach was a lymph node the size of a volleyball. His leg was completely . . . he couldn't even walk on it," Dank said.

After receiving the experimental treatment, the dog's cancer disappeared. He lived an additional two-and-a-half years. Based on the results of the dog trial, Efranat applied for approval in 2013 to run a human trial of the drug in Israel. Their plan was approved, and they began recruiting patients in the spring of 2014.

"It was unbelievable, those two dogs," Dank said.

———

By this point, I had soaked up plenty of enthusiasm from key players in comparative oncology — pet owners, veterinarians, and oncologists who were convinced that dogs might lead the way down new research paths that would bring hope to human patients. But what about the oncologists who weren't so deeply involved in research, but instead spent most of their time in the hospital trenches, laboring to keep their patients alive? I wondered if they thought dogs might help solve the endlessly unsolvable cancer puzzle. Or had they witnessed so much loss that they had no room for optimism?

Where better to look for answers, I figured, than with Dan Aderka, who managed Beth's treatment plan before and after her surgery? Aderka was a professor at Tel Aviv University and an oncologist who specialized in treating gastric, colon, and pancreatic cancer.

Unlike the surgeon and other doctors who whipped in and out of Beth's life — including the one who so cruelly called her an "experiment" after the radical surgery she had undergone did not work — Aderka stayed with Beth from beginning to end, choosing her medications, answering her questions, trying along with the rest of us to give her hope.

So shortly before I left for Israel, I sent Aderka an e-mail explaining that I was Beth's sister and I would appreciate meeting with him to tell him about all the dogs I had met who are helping cancer researchers. He agreed.

I had never encountered Aderka when I visited Beth during her treatments. Interacting with her doctors wasn't my role as the little sister, after all. I was there to try to keep her mind off the side effects of chemo, to help with the mountains of laundry produced by her four children, and to take my teenage niece shopping at the mall when Beth was too sick to leave the house.

I wasn't exactly sure what I wanted from Aderka. I didn't

expect him to comfort me, or even to try to convince me that the outlook for gastric cancer patients is improving. I expected that he would not discuss the specifics of my sister's cancer because of his obligation to protect patient privacy. But I did want to thank him for trying to cure her, mostly because I knew that during that terrible year of chemo and surgery and false hope, Beth hadn't found much room for gratitude.

So as our time in Israel was drawing to a close, Harry and I went to Aderka's home office in an upscale apartment building on a tree-lined street near Tel Aviv. As we walked up to the front door, I froze in a panic. I realized Aderka hadn't given me his apartment number, and all the names on the mailboxes outside the building were in Hebrew.

Harry and I started sounding out the names on the boxes, running our fingers from right to left along the cryptic, ancient lettering, calling up the distant lessons we had learned as seventh graders at Hebrew school in the 1970s.

"AH-DER-KAH," Harry said, pumping his fist triumphantly. "Apartment three!"

Harry went off to read in a nearby park, while I nervously went inside to meet Beth's oncologist. One flight up, I found the apartment and rang the bell.

Aderka opened the door and shook my hand. He was no taller than I, dressed in casual pants and a striped purple and blue shirt, with a gray goatee and glasses. As he showed me to a seat, my eyes were drawn to the figurines of the three wise monkeys, who hear, see, and speak no evil, perched on a bookshelf that was overflowing with textbooks on cancer. It was as if they were strategically placed there to give his desperately ill patients a bit of comic relief. I wondered if my sister had sat in this same chair, gazing at those monkeys, and if they had made her smile, even for a moment.

When I asked what made him choose this path — this specialty filled with the sheer horror of three largely incurable cancers — Aderka told me that he started his career as a family practitioner in the 1980s, but quickly grew bored.

"Internal medicine was . . . empty," he said, gesturing widely as he talked, and pausing often to find the right words, as if he were in front of a class of med students, eager to impart the right message. "I thought I could help much more in oncology. Now I view medicine through a specialty that includes everything: psychology — because you have to support families — and a lot of science, clinical decisions, cardiology, hematology. Everything. I find in oncology internal medicine at its best."

I admired Aderka for his ability to find fulfillment in treating patients who were facing such lousy prognoses. Stage four pancreatic cancer, best-case scenario for five-year survival based on both surgery options and location of the cancer: 16 percent.[7] Stage four colon cancer: 11 percent.[8] Gastric cancer, stage four, post-surgery — the sorry scenario my sister found herself facing: 4 percent survival.[9]

Aderka tried to explain the challenge of treating patients like Beth. "In gastric cancer, we may have one formula for starting treatment. Then we learn every tumor is different. Even one tumor in the same patient is different — if you take biopsies from different parts of the tumor, you'll find different mutations. Everyone has a new mutation. This is why, for the moment, we fail."

Before my sister started her first chemotherapy treatment, she had been determined to overcome the disease. She sent me an e-mail when she got back from that first treatment and was still in the twenty-four-hour respite period that happens between the infusion of chemo and the onslaught of side effects. She seemed well prepared for the horror to come.

"Waiting for the 'real' symptoms to kick in," she wrote. "I'm optimistic and ready to face whatever challenges come my way. I don't want the outside world to relate to me as a 'sick' person."

Beth planned to maintain as much of a normal routine as possible for the sake of her kids, she added.

"I've set off on the long road to recovery."

Then, silence.

For the next week, Beth did not answer her phone or her e-mails. She was so ill, I learned later, she could barely get out of bed. The sister I knew — the cheerful girl who grew into a gentle mother, handling the daily ups and downs of raising four children with loving patience — was gone forever. Hopeful words like "optimistic" and "recovery" vanished from her vocabulary.

When I visited Beth during her third round of chemotherapy, I watched her struggle to take the chemo pill that had been added to her treatment plan at the last minute — the "new" pill that was a fifty-year-old drug in a new, convenient package. It looked harmless: a baby-pink tablet no bigger than a Tylenol. But Beth knew, and I knew, that little pill packed the power to kill every cell in her body that resembled a cancer cell, even the non-cancerous ones that maintained everyday processes in her body and made her feel healthy and normal.

Beth took a deep breath, swallowed the pill with a glass of water, then grabbed a half-full glass of wine from the kitchen table and took a swig. She lacked the appetite or patience to sit down and eat dinner with her family, but she allowed herself that one mouthful of wine, that one small moment of pleasure, to take her mind off the coming nightmare of toxic side effects.

Beth told me she tried to imagine the chemo pill speeding its way to the tumor and obliterating it, as Aderka had urged her to do. Usually it didn't make her feel much better, but she trusted her doctor's advice and did it anyway, she said — a tiny gesture, but one that I took as a sign that my sister was holding on to some semblance of hope.

Beth's cancer nightmare engulfed her family, including their dog, Honey, whose various demands quickly became too much for my sister to handle. Despite Aderka's advice that she should get out and walk as much as possible, Beth was too exhausted to let Honey pull her down the street, or even to get up and open the door every time the dog wanted to go out back. So, shortly after Beth started her chemo treatments, the family gave Honey away to friends.

After six rounds of chemo, Beth checked into the hospital for the surgery, which would end up turning into a day-long marathon. But no one could guarantee that, even if all the cancer was removed, it wouldn't come back.

I called Beth the night before her surgery, and all she could do was cry and ask "Why me?"

I did not have an answer.

———

I asked Aderka if he believed dogs could help answer the questions that had plagued cancer researchers for centuries.

Aderka agreed that the usual animal models used for cancer research — the mice and rats that had human tumors implanted under their skin, or were somehow genetically engineered to mimic the human cancer experience — had failed to produce any significant advances. He recalled that Judah Folkman, the famed cancer researcher who discovered that some tumors could be eradicated by choking off their blood supply, had once said, jokingly, "If you are a mouse, we can take good care of you."

Aderka told me he was often frustrated by the complete disconnect between cancer science and the life-and-death battle oncologists face every day.

"Cancer models can seduce you into thinking they're real life," he said. "If you cure a mouse, it's not real."

He stopped short of hailing the dog as the solution to that problem, though.

"Models help us," he said. "But we treat human beings, not mice or dogs."

Aderka said that many of the newest drugs approved to treat cancer were not much of an improvement over what was already on the market. He was stunned, he said, when the FDA approved a drug to treat pancreatic cancer after the company that invented it demonstrated it improved survival by only twelve days.

"It costs $3,000 to $4,000 a month," Aderka said. "If I tell a patient, 'I can add twelve days to your life,' what is he going to think of me? Pharma tries to convince us that these drugs are much better. This is what the media hears and then transfers. They transfer hope."

I asked Aderka what he thought it would take to produce a breakthrough in cancer.

"I don't believe a breakthrough will be seen in the next twenty years," he said. "I'm terribly sorry to say that. I would like to see it. I'm sixty now. I don't think I'll see it. It's too complicated."

I started to wonder if Aderka saved all his positive thinking for his patients and kept none for himself.

"You must be hopeful about something," I said.

"You want something with hope? Something that's not skeptical?" he said. "Yes, I must see something hopeful. But at this moment I'm skeptical. Hope is a need. It's like, how do you say it, people sell hope as a . . ." Aderka paused to find the right word. "A product — hope is a product. It's not a necessity. You pay a lot for this good called hope."

"Thank you for taking care of my sister," I said as I packed up my notebook and stood up to leave. "It didn't work out for us, but . . ."

"You can understand our limitations," Aderka said, eager to complete my thought. "Understand, we did everything that can be done. We cannot do a bit beyond that. Yet."

Part of me was crushed Aderka didn't share my enthusiasm for dogs and their role in cancer research. Still, in

Aderka's final word to me, "yet," I detected a hint of optimism. No, he might not witness a cancer breakthrough in his lifetime. But with that small "yet," he seemed to be saying that I might see a cure in mine. Or perhaps Beth's children would see it in theirs.

"Yet" gave me hope.

Chapter 11
Banking on a Cure for Gastric Cancer

It was quite soon after I discovered comparative oncology that I first wondered, do dogs get stomach tumors? And if they do, could they serve as models for the scientists looking for cures for the disease that had taken Beth's life? When I fired up Google and typed "dogs," "gastric cancer," "comparative oncology," one name kept popping up in the search results: Elizabeth McNiel, who at the time was a veterinarian at Michigan State University.

McNiel was assembling a database of dogs who had gastric carcinomas — the same tumor type that had taken my sister's life. Her goal was to collect tumor samples from thousands of afflicted dogs around the United States and examine them for genetic clues to the disease — mutations, perhaps, or other out-of-the-ordinary gene signatures.

I called McNiel. She seemed surprised a journalist was interested in her project. Then I told her about my loss.

"What a devastating disease," she said, in an empathetic tone that comforted me. "Unfortunately in dogs, gastric cancer behaves just like the human disease does."

As she told me about all the dogs she had treated for gastric cancer, I thought she could have just as well been describing Beth's experience with the disease. The drugs available to treat stomach tumors aren't very effective in dogs, McNiel said. Surgeries to remove the cancer rarely work. It all sounded so depressingly familiar.

More than a year later — after my visits to veterinary schools around the country and my meeting with Beth's oncologist had left me hopeful about the future of cancer research — I decided to meet McNiel and learn more about how she and her patients might contribute to the world's understanding of gastric cancer.

By this time, McNiel had started a new job at Tufts University in Boston. She had taken her gastric cancer project with her and was continuing to collect tumor samples from dogs to study them. She split her time between two Tufts campuses: the Molecular Oncology Research Institute at the university's downtown medical center and the Cummings School of Veterinary Medicine a short drive away, in Grafton, Massachusetts.

I met McNiel at the medical campus in the heart of Boston's bustling Chinatown neighborhood. She took me to lunch at an Asian restaurant down the street from her lab, and invited along her colleague, Philip Hinds, professor of radiation oncology at the medical school. Over noodle soup, Hinds told me Tufts had set out to hire a veterinarian to work both at its medical school and veterinary school because the university wanted to boost its efforts in comparative oncology. They had wooed McNiel specifically because of her interest in gastric cancer.

Most of the more than 950,000 new gastric cancer cases diagnosed each year worldwide are concentrated in Asian countries such as Korea, Japan, and China.[1] Tufts' medical school, which has been located in Chinatown since 1949,[2] has long been devoted to giving back to the community around it, Hinds told me. That's why hunting for the causes and potential cures for gastric cancer was one of its top priorities. Hinds wanted to enhance those efforts with the knowledge McNiel was gaining by studying the disease in dogs, he said.

"She becomes a bridge between those research efforts," Hinds said.

One of the main reasons there have been so few advances in gastric cancer is that so little is known about what causes it. Only one small subtype of the disease, called hereditary diffuse gastric cancer syndrome, runs in families,[3] and only GISTs and HER2 positive stomach tumors have mutations that have been well-defined. The vast majority of patients, including my sister, have adenocarcinomas — tumors that appear randomly, grow silently, and rarely make themselves known until they've spread to other organs.

I once tried to make my sister laugh by telling her that scientists might find all the answers to her disease in sushi. In fact, I was only half kidding. I had heard that researchers at Ben Gurion University in Israel were trying to find a link between the typical Asian diet and gastric cancer. As yet, they had found no such connection. The long-held suspicion that diets rich in pickled foods upped the probability of developing cancer had never been definitively proven, either.

Soon after my first Google search of the topic, I uncovered a study from 1978 that suggested dogs might be good allies in the search for answers about human gastric cancer. The researchers, both veterinarians at the Animal Cancer Center in New York, had found a two-to-one ratio of males to females in the dogs with one type of gastric adenocarcinoma and a seven-to-one male-female ratio in another — similar to the gender ratio found in people with the disease. In most of the dogs, the disease had spread by the time their owners brought them in to be evaluated, presenting a treatment challenge similar to that in people, who usually don't detect symptoms until the disease is in stage four, when it is nearly impossible to cure. The researchers suggested that understanding the manner in which gastric cancer spreads in dogs could help oncologists better understand the disease and predict its course in people.[4]

McNiel told me she first became interested in gastric cancer when she was completing her veterinary degree at Texas A&M in the early 1990s. That was when the genomics revolution had started to uncover a number of genes that seemed to play a role in the development of cancer. At the same time, McNiel was noticing an odd trend in the oncology clinic where she was working.

"I didn't see stomach cancer very often in the oncology clinic, but it seemed like I was seeing it in Chow Chows more frequently," McNiel said. "So we looked at some veterinary databases and established that Chow Chows have about a twentyfold increased risk of developing stomach cancer."

Gastric cancer is so rare in dogs it accounts for less than 1 percent of all reported malignancies.[5] But it is highly concentrated in a small handful of breeds. In addition to Chow Chows, the disease is commonly reported in Belgian shepherds, such as Tervurens, and in collies.[6] McNiel also saw cases of the disease showing up in Keeshonds, Irish setters, Norwegian elkhounds, and Scottish terriers, she said.

By the time I met her, McNiel had collected 865 tissue samples from dogs, about a quarter of which were stomach tumors. The rest were normal stomach tissues donated by the owners of deceased pets. Her plan was to compare the healthy DNA to the cancerous DNA, in the hopes of finding genetic markers that were common in gastric tumors, she said.

"I think it will be hard to make sense of [gastric cancer] until we know the gene, or the genes, that predispose. And there may be more than one," McNiel said. "And there may be a different one for every breed. My gut is that there's something that all of them share."

McNiel told me that most of the dogs she had seen with gastric cancer were breeds known for having thick, fluffy coats.

"Is there something about being a fluffy dog that makes them predisposed? That may be the case," she said. "I mean, sometimes when we're breeding for particular traits, we're also picking up something that's undesirable in the genome that lies in close proximity to those traits."

McNiel, a bespectacled vet with short reddish hair and an approachable manner, had wide-ranging research interests. When I met her, she was also managing studies in feline oral squamous cell carcinoma and canine bladder cancer. But it was solving the mystery of gastric cancer that consumed much of her time and mental energy.

Among the dogs in McNiel's gastric cancer registry was Elton, a Keeshond owned by Michigan resident Roseanne Vorce. Elton was a medium-sized dog with a fox-like face and a double-layered, silver-and-black coat that framed his head like a lion's mane. The Keeshond (pronounced KAYZ-hawnd) breed is famed for its ability to master agility — the sport that requires dogs to leap over hurdles, scurry through tunnels, and weave between poles. Vorce trained Elton in the sport when he was a puppy, but he made it clear early on that competing wasn't his passion.

"He just wanted to be a homebody," Vorce said. "He was a sweet dog who just wanted to hang out. So one day I told him he didn't have to do agility anymore."

Training Elton in agility was all the more difficult because the dog often stopped in his tracks and regurgitated meals or treats he had eaten hours earlier. His vet didn't think much of it and prescribed the dog a standard heartburn remedy. Then, when Elton was two, he started vomiting daily.

Vorce, a trained pathologist who had spent part of her career working in the pharmaceutical industry, imagined the worst. Her other Keeshond, Julian, had just died of stomach cancer at age ten. Panicked, Vorce called the breeder who had sold her both dogs.

"She told me that she had to put down Elton's mother at age five," Vorce said. "She had stomach cancer."

After Elton's vets did exploratory surgery, they gave Vorce a diagnosis that was both hopeful and frustrating. Elton had lymphoplasmacytic gastritis — a general inflammation of the stomach that his vets thought might be pre-cancerous.

"They basically said, 'This is what we found. We don't know what it means.'"

Oncology researchers have long suspected there is a link between inflammation and cancer, but the effort to elucidate that connection has been fraught with false leads, contradictions, and questions that when answered raised more questions. In people, for example, a bug called Helicobacter pylori (H. pylori) has been shown to cause most ulcers and is now estimated to be a factor in 78 percent of all gastric cancer cases.[7] But being infected with the bacterium also decreases the risk of developing other cancers, including a type of stomach tumor that forms at the top of the organ, near the esophagus.[8]

Furthermore, a huge proportion of the general population is infected with H. pylori, but most people who have the bug never get ulcers or cancer.[9] No one knows why.

Dogs are not susceptible to H. pylori, McNiel explained to me. Nor do they get a mutation in a gene called E-cadherin, which is commonly linked to the familial form of gastric cancer in people. So she knew her tissue bank represented a huge fishing expedition — a place to search for answers without quite knowing what the questions should be.

As for Vorce, Elton's unclear diagnosis made her feel like she was caring for a dog whose health was a ticking time bomb.

"I was just waiting for him to develop symptoms," she said.

For the next eight years, Elton continued taking his heartburn pills and seemed to be doing fine. He occasionally had an upset stomach and refused to eat a meal, but he bounced back quickly, Vorce said. Then, just after he turned ten in the summer of 2013, Elton stopped eating.

"He wouldn't eat his kibble, but he would eat canned dog food," Vorce said. "Then he wouldn't eat canned dog food, but he'd eat scrambled eggs. Then he wouldn't eat that. I would just keep trying more and more tantalizing things."

Vorce had seen these symptoms before. When Julian was sick, she used to set her alarm for 2:30 a.m. every day and feed him some crackers to try to ease his nausea. She tried chemo, but it only bought Julian an extra three months of life. As Elton continued to turn his nose up as his favorite foods, Vorce resigned herself to the reality of what was wrong with him.

"I just knew it was stomach cancer."

Her veterinarian confirmed her suspicion. Vorce spent much of her spare time online looking for answers about what might be causing gastric cancer in this breed that she loved so much. She ran across an article about McNiel's research, but was shocked to see that it didn't mention Keeshonds. So she sent McNiel an e-mail.

"I told her I think there's a problem with this breed."

McNiel wrote right back to tell her she would absolutely welcome samples from Keeshonds. So after Elton died in September 2013, Vorce contributed samples of his stomach tumor to McNiel's study. Then she started encouraging members of her local breed club to do the same.

"There's a lot of resistance," she said. "Some pet owners don't want anyone cutting up their dog, whereas I'm a scientist. I'm thinking, 'My dog is gone. If it can help someone else, I'll give them anything.'"

I asked Vorce if losing two dogs to the same disease would make her shy away from the Keeshond breed in the future.

"I considered getting a different breed. However, the Keeshond has my heart," she replied. "Elton just got a bad deal genetically. He got a bad hand."

I couldn't help thinking of Beth when Vorce talked about Elton's bad fortune. "I was dealt a bad hand," Beth often said while fighting her disease. Indeed, and it was a bad hand that scientists were still far from being able to prevent.

—

Tufts' veterinary school in North Grafton, forty miles east of Boston, is part of a serene 594-acre campus of two-story brick buildings perched on green, rolling hills. When I arrived, two vets were walking a horse around the parking lot of the large-animal clinic, and pet owners were coming and going from the Foster Hospital for Small Animals, which treats twenty-six thousand dogs and cats per year.[10]

This campus is also home to the Tufts Wildlife Clinic, where students care for sick and injured New England wildlife — foxes, loons, and other creatures from the surrounding forests and waterways that are brought to the school by concerned locals. About sixteen hundred wild animals are admitted to Tufts each year, where veterinarians and students treat them and then release them, when possible, back into the wild.[11]

About four hundred students attend the Cummings Veterinary School, where comparative research is one of the primary pursuits. The school enrolls animals in clinical trials covering a dozen research areas, including behavior, nutrition, and orthopedics. And it isn't just dogs and cats who benefit from the research. During my visit, I learned that faculty and students were planning trials in squamous cell carcinoma in pet birds, as well as the pituitary disorder Cushing's disease in horses.

I sat down with John Berg, a professor of veterinary surgery, who told me that his comparative research included testing a new imaging technology developed by scientists at Duke University and the Massachusetts Institute of Technology. The machine was designed to help surgeons better see tumor cells, so they could be certain they were removing all of them during surgery.

"You would think, well can't you just tell? And the answer is you actually can't," Berg said. "That little bit of tissue you see right there that looks like it's not quite normal may be cancer, but it's often difficult to know if it is or not."

The company formed for the purpose of commercializing the technology developed a drug-device combo that would cause all the tumor cells to light up when viewed on a computer monitor in the operating room. In dogs,

Berg said, the technology was very reliable at catching cancer cells that might have otherwise been left behind. After Tufts ran a small trial in dogs, the company launched human clinical trials in breast cancer and sarcoma at Duke.

A second company was recruiting dogs at Tufts to test a different kind of imaging technology — a contrast material that, when used with a device such as a CT scan, distinguished between benign liver nodules and cancerous tumors. If it worked, Berg said, it might someday help patients avoid having to endure invasive biopsies.

As was the case with all of the veterinary schools I visited, Tufts was struggling to raise enough funds to meet all its goals in comparative oncology. To compile her gastric cancer collection, McNiel had received $70,000 in grants from the American Kennel Club's Canine Health Foundation. But to do a complete genomic analysis of the samples she had collected — to figure out which genes were turning on or off in the formation of stomach tumors — she needed more money.

"Getting the data set we need to be able to characterize the disease genetically and then figure out how it compares to humans is complicated and painstakingly slow," McNiel said. When she started studying this problem, she thought in a year or two she'd know what the gene is that predisposes dogs — and likely people — to gastric cancer, she said. "Now it looks like I'll be spending most of my career figuring out what the gene is."

McNiel had one of the leading geneticists working in comparative oncology on her side: Elaine Ostrander, head of the comparative genetics unit of the National Human

Genome Research Institute. Ostrander developed the Canine Genome Project, which was working to identify and map genetic markers of inherited canine diseases. She mapped the genes of several canine cancers that are similar in people, including bladder cancer and a rare disease called malignant histiocytosis. Ostrander was working with McNiel to help map gastric cancer in dogs.

McNiel was also grateful for donations she had received from people whose dogs had died from gastric cancer or who had healthy dogs that were at risk of the disease because of their breed.

"Of the healthy dogs, about 20 to 30 percent go on to develop some kind of cancer," she said. "And probably about 10 to 15 percent of those are gastric cancers, which actually suggests that gastric cancer is a lot more common even than we originally thought."

Databases such as McNiel's, which are commonly referred to as "cancer registries," are rare in veterinary medicine, but their value has already been well proven in human medicine. Cancer registries in the United States began to take off in 1956, when the American College of Surgeons started to encourage hospitals to record results of cancer treatment regimens and use that data to better understand the disease and determine the most effective treatment plans.[12] In Canada, a national registry was started in 1969. Today, the Canadian Cancer Registry collects and makes available data on all residents, alive or dead, who have been diagnosed with cancer since 1992.[13] Registries have become far more sophisticated over time, incorporating tissue samples, genomics data, and online platforms that make it easy for physicians and patients to find and participate in registry data-gathering.

In 2012, the American Society of Clinical Oncology (ASCO) — one of the world's largest societies of oncologists — began developing what the organization's chief medical officer, Richard L. Schilsky, told me was the ultimate cancer registry. The system, called CancerLinQ, was designed to allow any oncologist anywhere to record the details of what treatment regimens they were trying for various patients. The data would all be anonymous, and the registry would use rapid-learning technology to aggregate the experiences of patients all over the world. That would allow oncologists to search for patterns — common characteristics and experiences — to guide them in selecting the best treatments for their patients.

"It's a mechanism, essentially, to be in touch with every patient, and then to use that new knowledge to try to improve the quality of care for all patients with cancer," Schilsky said. "We anticipate over time we'll accumulate the records of millions of patients. These records will then also be a rich source of information for all sorts of observational studies that we hope will provide insights into the optimal treatments for different groups of individuals."

When I suggested that veterinarians should be able to use CancerLinQ, too, so they can apply the insights from treating human patients toward improving the care of pets, Schilsky agreed.

Schilsky is a gastroenterologist who has seen the devastation of gastric cancer up close. I told him about McNiel's gastric cancer registry and asked him if he could imagine someday that oncologists would gain insights from dogs to improve their treatments of people with gastric cancer.

"Knowledge is power, right?" he said. "Creating registries like this will allow veterinarians to understand the incidence of the problem, the prevalence of the problem, the characteristics of the dogs who get gastric cancer, and the outcomes of those animals. They will certainly learn something important."

When McNiel isn't studying gastric tumors or treating pets at Tufts, she is often traveling to breed clubs around the country to educate them about the cancer risk in their dogs and answer questions about what veterinary research was uncovering about the disease.

"I think the people in these clubs feel guilty about the fact that they may be breeding dogs that have a susceptibility to cancer," she said. "They just really want to figure out what's going on, so that they can breed healthier dogs."

I wondered if McNiel ever lost hope in her mission to find the clues that might lead to better cures for gastric cancer. Surely, she was devastated by the realization that what she expected to be a year-long search for the culprit gene might actually take her entire career. I thought it must be difficult for her to stand up in front of breed clubs and tell their members she still didn't know why their pets were so susceptible to gastric cancer, or to try to comfort families whose beloved pets were dying of this devastating disease long before their time should have run out.

But I didn't see devastation or disappointment in McNiel's eyes. I saw excitement for the scientific quest and certainty that she would find what she had set out to discover.

"How optimistic are you that more causes of gastric cancer and better treatments might happen in your career?" I asked.

"I'm an oncologist, so I'm naturally optimistic," she replied. "I think that if we can identify a gene — which I'm pretty determined to do — we'll get there."

As I left Tufts that day, I thought back to when I first heard the owners of Fawn — the cross-eyed sheltic who did so well in the first Palladia trial — say, "We believe in science," and realized how much my own attitude had changed about the power of science. I was feeling hopeful.

For the countless cancer patients who ask "Why me?" I wish I had an answer. I don't. But I'm optimistic that science is slowly unlocking the mysteries of this terrible disease. And I believe that the Fawns and Basils and Eltons of the world — the growing pack of dogs that have contributed to cancer research — offer new hope that scientists will develop better ways to detect cancer early, to improve our understanding of the disease, and ultimately, to find new cures.

Epilogue
I Believe in Science

As I completed this book, awareness of comparative oncology — and more broadly the importance of animal health — seemed to be exploding all around me.

Not surprisingly, Cheryl London at Ohio State was in the vanguard of the effort to bring attention to this field of research. In the fall of 2014, the university had more than eight oncology studies underway, and in September it announced to the press the first new therapy for canine lymphoma in two decades — Verdinexor, the Karyopharm drug that the FDA had made available to pet owners for limited use while the company completed the necessary trials for full approval. Karyopharm was also making progress on the human version of the drug.

"It's a real testament to where we are with integrating technology, information transfer, and translational science," London said in the press release. "It's the blueprint for how we can make drug discovery more efficient and successful."[1]

The other universities featured in this book were also planning more comparative oncology trials and making great headway in the research they had told me about when I visited them. For example, by the summer of 2014, Karin Sorenmo at the University of Pennsylvania had raised additional funds and resumed recruiting dogs for the mammary tumor research program. She had treated 120 dogs so far. There were plenty of stops and starts, but each time she thought she was running out of money, she told me, another donation came in and she was able to rescue more shelter dogs with mammary tumors. She and her Princeton research partner, Olga Troyanskaya, were preparing their first publication from the study.

As awareness of the value of comparative oncology grows, more and more human-oncology organizations are joining the effort. In the spring of 2014, researchers at the University of Kansas Medical Center and Children's Mercy Hospital in Kansas City teamed up with veterinarians at Colorado State to screen thousands of drug compounds against cell lines taken from both children and dogs with osteosarcoma. They called it a tournament of drugs — a massive, multi-discipline effort to figure out, with the help of dogs, which therapies are most likely to work against the disease.[2]

The Morris Animal Foundation's Golden Retriever Lifetime Health Project — the study managed by Rod Page at Colorado State University — reached its enrollment goal of three-thousand dogs by February 2015.

Meanwhile, the animal health industry is growing rapidly, and as a result, raising capital that may well benefit comparative oncology. In January 2013, Zoetis — the company created from the Pfizer unit that developed Palladia — raised a staggering $2.2 billion in a Wall Street initial public offering (IPO). That success encouraged several other animal-health start-ups to follow Zoetis's paw prints to Wall Street, including Aratana Therapeutics, which hauled in more than $125 million in two public stock offerings.

All of these newly wealthy companies, and several more privately held firms, are working enthusiastically at the intersection of human and animal health. Aratana is a good example. In March 2014, it licensed an experimental osteosarcoma treatment from a company called Advaxis, which was originally developing its compounds for people only. Advaxis sponsored a trial in pet dogs at the University of Pennsylvania's veterinary school, the results of which were so encouraging Aratana jumped in to develop the product for dogs, plus three other drugs in Advaxis's pipeline that looked promising. It was a win-win partnership: Advaxis was able to hand over the veterinary responsibilities to Aratana, but it would still be able to gain from the insights gathered from dogs to improve its efforts on the human side.

"We're getting out ahead of human medicine," Aratana CEO Steven St. Peter told me. "Obviously a human company wants high-quality data in dogs because that helps them move forward in humans."

For several years following the regulatory approvals of Palladia and Oncept, they were the only two drugs on the market specifically for pets with cancer. Now that's changing very rapidly, much to the benefit of pets and veterinarians. By early 2015, Aratana had one full approval and one conditional approval from the USDA for two different drugs to treat lymphoma.

These drugs are examples of a growing trend in animal health to take successful human products and transform them for use in dogs and cats — comparative oncology in reverse, if you will. Aratana's two products were inspired by drugs known as human monoclonal antibodies, which are effective in people but can't be used in dogs because they contain human proteins that would cause dangerous immune responses. So scientists "caninized" them, building them from dog antibodies instead. Several other companies are now working on canine monoclonal antibodies, and a handful are developing feline monoclonal antibodies, too.

Immunotherapy continues to revolutionize oncology, and by 2015, modified T cell transplantation such as the procedure tried in dogs with lymphoma at MD Anderson had become one of the most hotly pursued areas of cancer research. In January 2014, MD Anderson formed a three-year collaboration with pharmaceutical giant Johnson & Johnson to develop immunology treatments, which included supporting further research in T cell biology.[3] Several other research collaborations have formed around T cell transplants, including a partnership between the University of Pennsylvania and Novartis, who announced in late 2014 that two pilot studies of their personalized T cell therapy achieved a 90 percent remission rate in children and adults with leukemia.[4]

One of the early corporate supporters of comparative oncology, Aladár Szalay of Genelux, retired from his post as CEO in May 2014, before the company's virus-based therapies for dogs and people had made it through the development process. He was replaced by biotech industry veteran Thomas Zindrick, who told me when we spoke by phone that the company's comparative trial had confirmed the promise of technology it was developing to "help inform the human path." The company was looking for a partner to help take the veterinary product through the development process, and he was excited to see the new interest in the animal health industry among investors.

There were also some personnel changes at the veterinary schools I visited. Theresa Fossum, who originally introduced me to the field of comparative oncology, moved from Texas A&M in January 2014 to Midwestern University, where she was named vice president of research and strategic initiatives and charged with helping open the institution's new veterinary school.

While the growing interest from drug companies in comparative oncology is certainly a positive development, the most innovative ideas will continue to come from academia, and those scientists are in need of support for their research. Several charitable foundations were founded to support research in animal health generally and comparative oncology specifically. Should you wish to contribute to the cause, I list those organizations in the following pages.

Elizabeth McNiel's funding from the AKC to build the canine gastric tumor registry at Tufts was not renewed, but she was able to continue her work thanks to private donations she received from people whose dogs had suffered from the disease. By the end of 2014, her database included tissue samples from 977 dogs, 220 of whom had gastric carcinomas. She continued to work with Elaine Ostrander at the National Human Genome Research Institute and together they were preparing their first two publications: one describing the clinical aspects of canine stomach cancer, and the other assessing whether there are subtypes of canine gastric tumors that correlate with subtypes recently discovered in people.

Sadly, some of the dogs I had the pleasure of meeting or hearing about during my travels to veterinary oncology clinics are no longer with us. They include Cali and Rini from Penn's mammary tumor study; Sunny Boy, who gained more than three years of life on the melanoma vaccine Oncept; and Maya, the golden retriever treated at Colorado State. Maya, it turns out, participated in several subsequent lymphoma trials and was given chemo treatments that added eighteen months to her life. Her owners, Danielle and Kyle Balogh, had been wishing that Maya would meet their first child. She did. Danielle told me they will be forever thankful for that and for the opportunity to contribute to a possible cure.

Acknowledgments

First and foremost, thanks to all the pet owners who volunteered their stories for this book. I appreciate your openness, your willingness to talk with me on the phone or take the time to drive long distances to meet me, and in many cases, your hospitality in welcoming me into your homes. Most of all, I thank you and your dogs (or cats) for participating in comparative oncology research. Although it may be hard to see anything positive in your cancer experience, please understand that your pets' contributions to the advancement of science will make a difference in the search for a cure.

A big thanks to all the veterinarians who took breaks from their often frantic schedules to meet with me. I quickly realized as I began researching this book that academic veterinarians are some of the busiest people on the planet. Their typical day includes treating patients, teaching veterinary students, managing clinical trials, preparing research for publication, writing research grant proposals . . . the list goes on and on. I was never quite sure how they found time to eat and sleep.

Yet they made time to patiently explain their research to me, give me tours of their veterinary clinics, introduce me to pet owners, and answer multiple follow-up e-mails from me when I needed to make sure I was correctly describing the science behind their work. I am eternally grateful.

Thanks to my agent, Renee Zuckerbrot, for recognizing the value of this topic and for helping me strike the right balance between the science, the dogs, and my personal cancer loss, as I developed a plan for telling the story of dogs in cancer research.

I also appreciate the work of Jack David and everyone at ECW Press who helped bring this book to life and who located the perfect editor for it, Dinah Forbes. Dinah's years of editing experience, combined with her love of dogs, proved invaluable for helping me get across how vital — and fascinating — this research is to our future health and that of our four-legged friends.

A special thanks to my husband, Harry, who read each chapter draft carefully and thoughtfully, providing invaluable insight as both a dog lover and a voracious reader with a keen interest in science. Thank you also for taking care of our dog, Molly, each time I jetted off to a veterinary school to complete the next stage of research.

Of course, I would be remiss if I didn't thank Molly. She has seen me through the illness and death of my sister, the meeting and marrying of my husband, and countless other ups and downs. Most mornings, Molly jumps on the bed as I'm waking up and puts her paw in my hand, as if to tell me how excited she is for us to start our day together. I highly recommend having a dog to hold your hand through life.

How You Can Help

If this book has inspired you to support comparative oncology research (and I hope it has), you will find a number of worthy organizations grateful to receive your donation. You can donate directly to the universities that are leading comparative oncology research, all of which are listed on the website of the Comparative Oncology Trials Consortium (ccrod.cancer.gov/confluence/display/ CCRCOPWeb/Home). There are also several independent foundations that support these trials. Some of these groups were founded by pet owners who had such positive experiences participating in comparative research with their dogs that they decided to give back by forming charitable foundations to support future trials. I have also included here several human cancer foundations, mostly organized according to the tumor types I focused on in this book.

Animal Health/
Comparative Oncology Foundations

Puppy Up Foundation (formerly 2 Million Dogs)
   www.2milliondogs.org

American Kennel Club Canine Health Foundation
   www.akcchf.org

Animal Cancer Foundation
   www.acfoundation.org

Animal Health Foundation
   www.animalhealthfoundation.net

Blue Buffalo Foundation for Cancer Research
   www.bluebuffalo.com/bbfcr

Gabriel Institute
   www.gabrielinstitute.org

InSitu Foundation
   www.dogsdetectcancer.org

Land of PureGold Foundation
   www.landofpuregold.com/cancer

Morris Animal Foundation
   www.morrisanimalfoundation.org

National Canine Cancer Foundation
   www.wearethecure.org

Perseus Foundation
   www.theperseusfoundation.org

Puccini Foundation
   www.puccinifoundation.org

Will-Power Cancer Research Fund
   www.modianolab.org/Will_Power.shtml

Veterinary Cancer Society
   www.vetcancersociety.org

Winn Feline Foundation
   www.winnfelinefoundation.org

Human Cancer Foundations

MELANOMA:

American Melanoma Foundation
 www.melanomafoundation.org
Melanoma Research Foundation
 www.melanoma.org
The Skin Cancer Foundation
 www.skincancer.org

OSTEOSARCOMA:

Sarcoma Foundation of America
 www.curesarcoma.org

LYMPHOMA:

Leukemia & Lymphoma Society
 www.lls.org
Lymphoma Research Foundation
 www.lymphoma.org

BREAST CANCER:

Breast Cancer Research Foundation
 www.bcrfcure.org
Canadian Breast Cancer Foundation
 www.cbcf.org
Susan G. Komen Foundation
 www.komen.org

GASTRIC CANCER:

Debbie's Dream Foundation
 www.debbiesdream.org
Gastric Cancer Foundation
 www.gastriccancer.org
No Stomach for Cancer
 www.nostomachforcancer.org

GENERAL:

American Cancer Society
    www.cancer.org
American Society of Clinical Oncology
    www.asco.org
Stand Up to Cancer
    www.standup2cancer.org

Learn More

If your pet has been diagnosed with cancer and you're looking for a clinical trial, or you'd just like to find out more
about comparative oncology, there are a lot of resources
out there to help you. Here's a list of helpful books, veterinary websites and clinics, and funding sources for pet
owners facing this difficult diagnosis.

Books

Demian Dressler, with Susan Ettinger. *The Dog Cancer Survival
Guide: Full Spectrum Treatments to Optimize Your Dog's Life
Quality & Longevity*. Maui: Maui Media, 2011.
www.dogcancerblog.com.

Laurie Kaplan. *Help Your Dog Fight Cancer: What Every
Caretaker Should Know about Canine Cancer*. 2nd ed. JanGen
Press, 2008. www.jangenpress.com.

Lola Ball. *When Your Dog Has Cancer: Making the Right*

Decisions for You and Your Dog. Dogwise Publishing, 2012.
www.whenyourdoghascancer.org.

Barbara Natterson-Horowitz, M.D., and Kathryn Bowers.
*Zoobiquity: The Astonishing Connection Between Human and
Animal Health.* New York: Vintage Books, 2012.
www.zoobiquity.com.

Jeremy R. Garrett, ed. *The Ethics of Animal Research:
Exploring the Controversy.* Cambridge: The MIT Press, 2012.
mitpress.mit.edu/books/ethics-animal-research.

Veterinary Oncology Clinical Trial Information

Comparative Oncology Trials Consortium
ccrod.cancer.gov/confluence/display/CCRCOPWeb/
Clinical+Trials

National Veterinary Cancer Registry
nationalveterinarycancerregistry.org

Veterinary Cancer Society
www.vetcancertrials.org

US Food & Drug Administration
"My Dog Has Cancer: What Do I Need to Know?"
www.fda.gov/ForConsumers/ConsumerUpdates/ucm412208.htm

Colorado State University Flint Animal Cancer Center
www.csuanimalcancercenter.org/clinical-trials

Cornell University College of Veterinary Medicine
www.vet.cornell.edu/faculty/hume/clinicaltrials.cfm

North Carolina State University College of Veterinary Medicine
www.cvm.ncsu.edu/ccmtr/onco.html

Purdue University College of Veterinary Medicine
www.vet.purdue.edu/orpd/clinical-trials.php

Texas A&M School of Veterinary Medicine and Biomedical Sciences
vetmed.tamu.edu/clinical-trials/canine-oncology

The Ohio State University College of Veterinary Medicine
vet.osu.edu/research/recruiting-clinical-trials

Tufts Cummings School of Veterinary Medicine
sites.tufts.edu/vetclinicaltrials/specialty/oncology

University of California Davis School of Veterinary Medicine
www.vetmed.ucdavis.edu/clinicaltrials/current_trials/by_
service/oncology.cfm

University of Georgia College of Veterinary Medicine
www.vet.uga.edu/research/clinical/current

University of Guelph Ontario Veterinary College
ovc.uoguelph.ca/icci

University of Illinois Veterinary Teaching Hospital
vetmed.illinois.edu/vth/services/clinical_trials.html

University of Minnesota College of Veterinary Medicine
www.cvm.umn.edu/cic/current/home.html

University of Missouri Scott Endowed Program in Veterinary Oncology
www.cvm.missouri.edu/oncology/current.html

University of Pennsylvania School of Veterinary Medicine
research.vet.upenn.edu/ClinicalStudies/tabid/4515/Default.aspx

University of Tennessee College of Veterinary Medicine
www.vet.utk.edu/studies/index.php

University of Wisconsin-Madison School of Veterinary
Medicine
uwveterinarycare.wisc.edu/clinical-studies/oncology

Washington State University College of Veterinary Medicine
vcs.vetmed.wsu.edu/research/clinical-studies

Funding Sources for Pet Owners Facing Cancer

Brown Dog Foundation, Inc.
www.browndogfoundation.org

The Dog and Cat Cancer Fund
www.dccfund.org

Fetch a Cure
www.fetchacure.org

Frankie's Friends
www.frankiesfriends.org

Magic Bullet Fund
www.themagicbulletfund.org

Paws 4 a Cure
www.paws4acure.org

The Pet Fund
www.thepetfund.com

Notes

Prologue

1   FDA, "First Drug to Treat Cancer in Dogs Approved," June 3, 2009, http://www.fda.gov/NewsEvents/Newsroom/PressAnnouncements/ucm164118.htm.

2   Cheryl A. London et al., "Phase I Dose-Escalating Study of SU11654, a Small Molecule Receptor Tyrosine Kinase Inhibitor, in Dogs with Spontaneous Malignancies," *Clinical Cancer Research* 9, no. 7 (July 2003): 2755-68.

3   Cheryl A. London et al., "Multi-center, Placebo-controlled, Double-blind, Randomized Study of Oral Toceranib Phosphate (SU11654), a Receptor Tyrosine Kinase Inhibitor, for the Treatment of Dogs with Recurrent (Either Local or Distant) Mast Cell Tumor Following Surgical Excision," *Clinical Cancer Research* 15 (June 2009): 3856-65.

Chapter 1

1   FDA, "FDA Issues Advice to Make Earliest Stages of Clinical Drug Development More Efficient," January 12, 2006, http://www.fda.gov/NewsEvents/Newsroom/PressAnnouncements/2006/ucm108576.htm.

2   Marlene Cimons, "Cancer Drugs Face Long Road from Mice to

Men," *Los Angeles Times*, May 6, 1998, http://articles.latimes
.com/1998/may/06/news/mn-46795.

3   Xose S. Puente et al., "Comparative analysis of cancer genes in the
    human and chimpanzee genomes," *BMC Genomics* 7, no. 15 (2006).

4   "NIH to Reduce Significantly the Use of Chimpanzees in Research,"
    June 26, 2013, http://www.nih.gov/news/health/jun2013/od-26.htm.

5   California Biomedical Research Association, "Fact Sheet: Primates in
    Biomedical Research," http://ca-biomed.org/pdf/media-kit/
    fact-sheets/fs-primate.pdf.

6   National Cancer Institute Center for Cancer Research, "Disease
    Information." https://ccrod.cancer.gov/confluence/display/
    CCRCOPWeb/Disease+Information.

7   Stefan Lovgren, "Dog Genome Mapped, Shows Similarities
    to Humans," *National Geographic News*, December 7, 2005,
    http://news.nationalgeographic.com/news/2005/12/1207_051207_
    dog_genome.html.

8   Adam R. Boyko, "The domestic dog: man's best friend in the
    genomic era," *Genome Biology* 12, no. 216 (2011),
    http://genomebiology.com/2011/12/2/216.

9   Albert T. Liao et al., "Inhibition of Constitutively Active Forms of
    Mutant Kit by Multitargeted Indolinone Tyrosine Kinase Inhibitors,"
    Blood 100, no. 8 (July 2002): 585-93.

10 Raymond M. Shaheen et al., "Tyrosine Kinase Inhibition of Multiple
    Angiogenic Growth Factor Receptors Improves Survival in Mice
    Bearing Colon Cancer Liver Metastases by Inhibition of Endothelial
    Cell Survival Mechanisms," *Cancer Research* 61, no. 4 (February
    2001): 1464-1468.

11 Cristiana Sessa et al., "Phase I clinical and pharmacological evaluation
    of the multi-tyrosine kinase inhibitor SU006668 by chronic oral
    dosing," *European Journal of Cancer* 42, no.2 (January 2006): 171-78.

12 Liao et al., "Inhibition of Constitutively Active Forms of Mutant Kit."

13 FDA, "FDA Approves New Treatment for Gastrointestinal and
    Kidney Cancer," January 26, 2006, http://www.fda.gov/NewsEvents/
    Newsroom/PressAnnouncements/2006/ucm108583.htm.

14 World Health Organization, International Agency for Research
    on Cancer, "Stomach Cancer Estimated Incidence, Mortality and
    Prevalence Worldwide in 2012,"

http://globocan.iarc.fr/Pages/fact_sheets_cancer.aspx.

15   National Cancer Institute, "SEER Stat Fact Sheets: Stomach Cancer,"
     http://seer.cancer.gov/statfacts/html/stomach.html.

16   Memorial Sloan Kettering Cancer Center, "About Stomach
     Cancer," http://www.mskcc.org/cancer-care/adult/stomach-gastric/
     about-stomach.

17   Cheryl A. London et al., "Phase I Dose-Escalating Study of su11654,
     a Small Molecule Receptor Tyrosine Kinase Inhibitor, in Dogs with
     Spontaneous Malignancies," *Clinical Cancer Research* 9, no. 7 (July
     2003): 2755-68.

18   Associated Press, "UC Davis School of Veterinary Loses Full
     Accreditation," December 4, 1998, http://articles.latimes.com/1998/
     dec/04/news/mn-50604.

19   Alice Villalobos, "Power of the Bond Reinvigorates UC Davis,"
     Veterinary Practice News, April 17, 2009,
     http://www.veterinarypracticenews.com/Vet-Practice-News-Columns/
     Bond-Beyond/Uc-Davis-School-Veterinary-Medicine.

20   UC Davis, *Veterinary Medicine News*, Spring 2005.

21   UC Davis, "About the Veterinary Medical Teaching Hospital,"
     http://www.vetmed.ucdavis.edu/vmth/about_vmth/index.cfm.

22   London et al., "Phase I."

23   Katherine G. Moss et al., "Hair Depigmentation Is a Biological
     Readout for Pharmacological Inhibition of KIT in Mice and
     Humans," *The Journal of Pharmacology and Experimental Therapeutics*
     307, no. 2 (November 2003): 476-80.

Chapter 2

1   The Ohio State University College of Veterinary Medicine, "About
    the College," http://vet.osu.edu/cvm/about-college.

2   Seiichi Hirota et al., "Gain-of-Function Mutations of c-kit in Human
    Gastrointestinal Stromal Tumors," *Science* 279 (January 1998): 577-80.

3   The Humane Society of the United States, "Success for Animals Used
    to Test Botox," July 8, 2011, http://www.humanesociety.org/issues/
    cosmetic_testing/ending_botox_testing/allergan_botox_test.html.

4   Cheryl A. London et al., "Multi-center, Placebo-controlled, Double-
    blind, Randomized Study of Oral Toceranib Phosphate (SU11654), a

Receptor Tyrosine Kinase Inhibitor, for the Treatment of Dogs with Recurrent (Either Local or Distant) Mast Cell Tumor Following Surgical Excision," *Clinical Cancer Research* 15 (June 2009): 3856-65.

5   Ibid.

6   Cheryl A. London et al., "Preclinical Evaluation of the Novel, Orally Bioavailable Selective Inhibitor of Nuclear Export (SINE) KPT-335 in Spontaneous Canine Cancer: Results of a Phase I Study," *PLoS One* 9, no. 2 (2014): 1-11.

7   Karyopharm Therapeutics, "Karyopharm Announces: FDA Considers the Effectiveness and Safety Technical Sections Complete to Support Conditional Approval for the New Animal Drug Application for Verdinexor (KPT-335) to Treat Lymphoma in Client Owned Dogs," June 16, 2014,
http://investors.karyopharm.com/releasedetail.cfm?releaseid=854785.

8   The Ohio State University Center for Clinical and Translational Science, "New Cancer Drug for Dogs Benefits Human Research, Drug Development," September 9, 2014,
http://www.newswise.com/articles/new-cancer-drug-for-dogs-benefits-human-research-drug-development.

9   Cheryl London et al., "Preliminary Evidence for Biologic Activity of Toceranib Phosphate (Palladia(®)) in Solid Tumours," *Veterinary Comparative Oncology* 10, no. 3 (September 2012): 194-205.

Chapter 3

1   American Cancer Society, "What Are the Key Statistics about Melanoma Skin Cancer?"
http://www.cancer.org/cancer/skincancer-melanoma/detailedguide/melanoma-skin-cancer-key-statistics.

2   National Canine Cancer Foundation, "Melanoma-Melanocytic Tumors," http://www.wearethecure.org/melanoma.

3   Philip J. Bergman and Jedd D. Wolchok, "Of Mice and Men (and Dogs): Development of a Xenogeneic DNA Vaccine for Canine Oral Malignant Melanoma," *Cancer Therapy* 6 (October 2008): 817-26.

4   Christopher R. Parish, "Cancer Immunotherapy: The Past, the Present and the Future," *Immunology and Cell Biology* 81, no. 2 (April 2003): 106-13.

5   Philip J. Bergman et al., "Long-Term Survival of Dogs with Advanced
     Malignant Melanoma after DNA Vaccination with Xenogeneic
     Human Tyrosinase: A Phase I Trial," *Clinical Cancer Research* 9, no. 4
     (April 2003): 1284-90.

6   L.A. Elsken et al., "Regulations for Vaccines Against Emerging
     Infections and Agrobioterrorism in the United States of America,"
     Scientific and Technical Review (International Office of Epizootics) 26,
     no. 2 (August 2007): 429-41.

7   Deborah A. Grosenbaugh et al., "Safety and Efficacy of a Xenogeneic
     DNA Vaccine Encoding for Human Tyrosinase as Adjunctive
     Treatment For Oral Malignant Melanoma in Dogs Following Surgical
     Excision of the Primary Tumor," *American Journal of Veterinary
     Research*, 72, vol. 12 (December 2011): 1631-38.

8   Ibid.

9   Merial, "Merial Receives Full License Approval for ONCEPT™
     Canine Melanoma Vaccine," February 16, 2010. http://us.merial
     .com/merial_corporate/news/press_releases/02-16-2010_ONCEPT_
     consumer_release.asp.

10   Jedd D. Wolchok et al., "Safety and Immunogenicity of Tyrosinase
     DNA Vaccines in Patients with Melanoma," *Molecular Therapy* 15,
     no. 11 (November 2007): 2044-50.

11   Stacey Oke, "Field Study for Equine Melanoma Vaccine Announced,"
     The Horse, September 21, 2014, http://www.thehorse.com/
     articles/34570/field-study-for-equine-melanoma-vaccine-announced.

Chapter 4

1   "How many people get osteosarcoma?" American Cancer Society,
     http://www.cancer.org/cancer/osteosarcoma/overviewguide/
     osteosarcoma-overview-key-statistics.

2   Malcolm A. Smith et al., "Outcomes for Children and Adolescents
     with Cancer: Challenges for the Twenty-First Century," *Journal of
     Clinical Oncology* 28, no.15 (May 2010): 2625-34.

3   Fabienne Mueller, Bruno Fuchs, and Barbara Kaser-Hotz,
     "Comparative Biology of Human and Canine Osteosarcoma,"
     Anticancer Research 27, no. 1A (January-February 2007): 155-64.

4   Melissa Paoloni et al., "Canine Tumor Cross-Species Genomics

Uncovers Targets Linked to Osteosarcoma Progression," *BMC Genomics* 10, no. 625 (December 2009).

5   I.D. Kurzman et al., "Adjuvant Therapy for Osteosarcoma in Dogs: Results of Randomized Clinical Trials Using Combined Liposome-Encapsulated Muramyl Tripeptide and Cisplatin," *Clinical Cancer Research* 1, no. 12 (December 1995): 1595-1601.

6   Paul A. Meyers et al., "Osteosarcoma: A Randomized, Prospective Trial of the Addition of Ifosfamide and/or Muramyl Tripeptide to Cisplatin, Doxorubicin, and High-Dose Methotrexate," *Journal of Clinical Oncology* 23, no. 9 (March 2005): 2004-11.

7   Colorado State University, "Veterinary Teaching Hospital Renovation," http://supporting.colostate.edu/vth-renovation/.

8   Colorado State University, "Flint Animal Cancer Center Biennial Report," February 2011, http://www.csuanimalcancercenter.org/assets/files/acc_biennial_report_2011.pdf.

9   Colorado State University, "Flint Foundation Gives $3 Million for Animal Cancer Center; Largest Cash Gift Ever to College of Veterinary Medicine," August 16, 2000, http://www.news.colostate.edu/Release/2020.

10 Jaime F. Modiano et al., "Inflammation, Apoptosis, and Necrosis Induced by Neoadjuvant Fas Ligand Gene Therapy Improves Survival of Dogs with Spontaneous Bone Cancer," *Molecular Therapy* 20, no. 12 (December 2012): 2234-43.

11 Ibid.

12 Roche, "FDA Approves Herceptin for HER2-Positive Metastatic Stomach Cancer," October 21, 2010, http://www.roche.com/media/media_releases/med-cor-2010-10-21.htm.

13 Noel R. Monks et al., "A Multi-Site Feasibility Study for Personalized Medicine in Canines With Osteosarcoma," *Journal of Translational Medicine* 11, no. 158 (July 2013), http://www.translational-medicine.com/content/11/1/158.

14 Jaime F. Modiano et al., "Neoadjuvant Fas Ligand Gene Therapy."

15 Takeda, "Takeda to Acquire IDM Pharma, Adding Mepact (Mifamurtide), The First Treatment Approved for Osteosarcoma in More Than 20 Years, to Its Oncology Franchise," May 18, 2009, http://www.takeda.com/news/2009/20090518_3701.html.

16 University of Texas MD Anderson Cancer Center, "When Discovery

Collides With Reality: The Journey of an Orphan Drug," *Children's Cancer Center Hospital Newsletter*, Spring 2013, http://www.mdanderson.org/publications/children s cancer hospital newsletter/issues/2013-spring/mepact.html.

17   Stephen J. Withrow and Ross M. Wilkins, "Crosstalk from Pets to People: Translational Osteosarcoma Treatments," *ILAR Journal*, 51, no. 3 (2010): 208-13.

Chapter 5

1   American Kennel Club Canine Health Foundation, "Canine Lymphoma," August 30, 2009. http://www.akcchf.org/canine-health/your-dogs-health/canine-lymphoma.html.

2   UC Davis, "Understanding Cancer in Golden Retrievers," http://www.vetmed.ucdavis.edu/CCAH/local-assets/pdfs/UnderstandingCancerinGoldenRetrievers2.pdf.

3   National Cancer Institute, "SEER Stat Fact Sheets: Non-Hodgkin Lymphoma," http://seer.cancer.gov/statfacts/html/nhl.html.

4   Purdue University, "Canine Lymphomas," http://www.vet.purdue.edu/pcop/canine-lymphoma-research.php.

5   American Cancer Society, "What Are the Risk Factors for Non-Hodgkin Lymphoma?" http://www.cancer.org/cancer/non-hodgkinlymphoma/detailedguide/non-hodgkin-lymphoma-risk-factors.

6   Framingham Heart Study, "History of the Framingham Heart Study," http://www.framinghamheartstudy.org/about-fhs/history.php.

7   Rainer Storb and E. Donnall Thomas, "The Scientific Foundation of Marrow Transplantation Based on Animal Studies," *Bone Marrow Transplantation*, Blackwell (1994): 3-11.

8   National Bone Marrow Donor Program, "National Bone Marrow Donor Program® and Be the Match® Key Messages, Facts & Figures," http://bethematch.org/News/Facts_and_Figures_(PDF)/.

9   Texas A&M, "Veterinary Medical Teaching Hospital (VMTH)," http://vetmed.tamu.edu/distinguishing-hallmarks/service.

10   Texas A&M, "New $120 Million Classroom Building Approved for Texas A&M College of Veterinary Medicine & Biomedical Sciences," http://vetmed.tamu.edu/news/press-releases/

new-$120-million-classroom-building-approved-for-texas-am-college-of-veterinary-medicine-biomedical-sciences#.uιιru2Q04b0.

11   Colleen M. O'Connor et al., "Adoptive T-cell therapy improves treatment of canine non–Hodgkin lymphoma post chemotherapy," *Scientific Reports* 2, no. 249 (February 2012), http://www.ncbi.nlm.nih.gov/pmc/articles/PMC3278154/.

12   Zoltán Ivics et al., "Molecular Reconstruction of Sleeping Beauty, a Tc1-like Transposon from Fish, and Its Transposition in Human Cells," *Cell* 91, no. 4 (November 1997): 501-10.

Chapter 6

1   MD Anderson Cancer Center, "Ductal Carcinoma In Situ," MD Anderson *OncoLog* 55, no. 1 (January 2010), http://www2.mdanderson.org/depts/oncolog/articles/10/1-jan/1-10-compass.html.

2   The Merck Veterinary Manual, "Overview of Mammary Tumors," http://www.merckmanuals.com/vet/reproductive_system/mammary_tumors/overview_of_mammary_tumors.html.

3   American Cancer Society, "Breast Cancer Facts & Figures 2011-2012," http://www.cancer.org/acs/groups/content/@epidemiology surveilance/documents/document/acspc-030975.pdf.

4   P. Rivera et al., "Mammary Tumor Development in Dogs Is Associated with BRCA1 and BRCA2," *Cancer Research* 69, no. 22 (November 2009), 8770–74.

5   American Cancer society, "What Are the Risk Factors for Breast Cancer?" http://www.cancer.org/cancer/breastcancer/detailedguide/breast-cancer-risk-factors.

6   VCA Animal Hospitals, "Mammary Tumors in Dogs — Benign," http://www.vcahospitals.com/main/pet-health-information/article/animal-health/mammary-tumors-in-dogs-benign/411.

7   Merck Veterinary Manual.

8   University of Pennsylvania, "Ryan Veterinary Hospital," http://www.vet.upenn.edu/veterinary-hospitals/ryan-veterinary-hospital.

9   University of Pennsylvania, "New Bolton Center," http://www.vet.upenn.edu/veterinary-hospitals/NBC-hospital.

10   K.U. Sorenmo et al., "Canine Mammary Gland Tumours; A Histological Continuum from Benign to Malignant; Clinical and

Histopathological Evidence," *Veterinary and Comparative Oncology* 7, no. 3 (September 2009): 162-72.

11   American Cancer Society, "Breast Cancer Survival Rates by Stage," http://www.cancer.org/cancer/breastcancer/detailedguide/breast-cancer-survival-by-stage.

12   American Cancer Society, "What Are the Survival Rates for Colorectal Cancer by Stage?" http://www.cancer.org/cancer/colonandrectumcancer/detailedguide/colorectal-cancer-survival-rates.

13   American Cancer Society, "Survival Rates for Stomach Cancer, by Stage," http://www.cancer.org/cancer/stomachcancer/detailedguide/stomach-cancer-survival-rates.

14   American Cancer Society, "Current Grants by Cancer Type as of March 1, 2015," http://www.cancer.org/research/currentlyfundedcancerresearch/grants-by-cancer-type.

15   National Institutes of Health, "Estimates of Funding for Various Research, Condition, and Disease Categories (RCDC)," http://report.nih.gov/categorical_spending.aspx.

16   National Football League, "About a Crucial Catch," http://www.nfl.com/pink.

Chapter 7

1   Elizabeth Kelly and Stephen J. Russell, "History of Oncolytic Viruses: Genesis to Genetic Engineering," *Molecular Therapy*, 15, no. 4 (2007): 651-59.

2   Ibid.

3   Stefan Riedel, "Edward Jenner and the History of Smallpox and Vaccination," *BUMC Proceedings* 18, no. 1 (January 2005): 21-5.

4   Mark S. Ferguson, Nicholas R. Lemoine, and Yaohe Wang, "Systemic Delivery of Oncolytic Viruses: Hopes and Hurdles," *Advances in Virology* 2012, no. 805629 (2012): 1-14.

5   Genelux, "Genelux Corporation Announces Ground-Breaking Clinical Study Evaluating Oncolytic Vaccinia Virus in Canine Cancer Patients," June 28, 2012, http://www.genelux.com/june-28-2012/.

6   Laura Adelmann, "A 'tail' of hope," SunThisWeek.com, August 1, 2013, http://sunthisweek.com/2013/08/01/a-tail-of-hope/.

7 M. Arendt, L. Nasir, and I.M. Morgan, "Oncolytic Gene Therapy for Canine Cancers: Teaching Old Dog Viruses New Tricks," *Veterinary and Comparative Oncology* 7, no. 3 (2009): 153–61.

8 Steven E. Suter et al., "In Vitro Canine Distemper Virus Infection of Canine Lymphoid Cells: A Prelude to Oncolytic Therapy for Lymphoma," *Clinical Cancer Research* 11, no. 4 (February 2005): 1579-87.

9 Helen L Del Puerto et al., "Canine Distemper Virus Induces Apoptosis in Cervical Tumor Derived Cell Lines," *Virology Journal* 8, no. 334 (June 2011), http://www.virologyj.com/content/8/1/334.

10 Amgen, "Amgen Presents New Data From Phase 3 Study of Talimogene Laherparepvec in Patients with Metastatic Melanoma," September 30, 2013, http://www.amgen.com/media/media_pr_detail.jsp?year=2013&releaseID=1859577.

11 Genelux, "Genelux Corporation Announces Treatment of First Patient in Phase I/II Clinical Trial of GL-ONC1 in Advanced Peritoneal Cavity Cancers," May 31, 2012, http://www.genelux.com/thursday-may-31-2012/.

12 National Institutes of Health, "Drug Record: Doxorubicin, Epirubicin, Idarubicin," http://livertox.nlm.nih.gov/DoxorubicinEpirubicinIdarubicin.htm.

13 National Institutes of Health, "Drug Record: Cisplatin," http://livertox.nlm.nih.gov/Cisplatin.htm.

14 National Institutes of Health, "Drug Record: Fluorouracil," http://livertox.nlm.nih.gov/Fluorouracil.htm.

Chapter 8

1 WebMD, "Infection and Tumors of the Breasts in Cats," excerpted from *Cat Owners Home Veterinary Handbook* (Wiley 2008) by Delbert Carlson and James M. Giffin, http://pets.webmd.com/cats/infection-tumors-breast-cancer-cats.

2 "Overview of Mammary Tumors," The Merck Manual Veterinary Edition, http://www.merckmanuals.com/vet/reproductive_system/mammary_tumors/overview_of_mammary_tumors.html.

3 Ontario Veterinary College, "History of OVC," http://ovc.uoguelph.ca/history.

4   Katrina R. Bauer et al., "Descriptive Analysis of Estrogen Receptor (ER)-Negative, Progesterone Receptor (PR)-Negative, and HER2-Negative Invasive Breast Cancer, the So Called Triple-Negative Phenotype," *Cancer* 109, no. 9 (May 2007): 1721-28.

5   Joan U. Pontius et al., "Initial Sequence and Comparative Analysis of the Cat Genome," *Genome Research* 17, no. 11 (November 2007): 1675-89.

6   Stephen J. O'Brien et al., "The Feline Genome Project," *Annual Review of Genetics* 36 (June 2002). 657-06.

7   William D. Hardy, Jr., et al., "Biology of Feline Leukemia Virus in the Natural Environment," *Cancer Research* 36 (February 1976), 582-588.

8   Susan M. Cotter et al., "Multiple Cases of Feline Leukemia and Feline Infectious Peritonitis in a Household," *Journal of the American Veterinary Medical Association*, 162, no. 12 (July 1973): 1054-8.

9   Dawn D. Bennett, "Vaccine for Cats' Number One Killer," *Science News*, February 16, 1985, http://www.thefreelibrary.com/ Vaccine+for+cats'+number+one+killer.-a03645279.

10 C.J. Bailey and C. Day, "Metformin: Its Botanical Background," *Practical Diabetes International*, 21, no. 3 (April 2004), 115-7, http://onlinelibrary.wiley.com/doi/10.1002/pdi.606/epdf.

11 Matteo Monami et al., "Metformin and Cancer Occurrence in Insulin-Treated Type 2 Diabetic Patients," *Diabetes Care* 34, no. 1 (January 2011), 129-31.

12 Ibid.

13 F.P. Kuhajda, "AMP-activated Protein Kinase and Human Cancer: Cancer Metabolism Revisited," *International Journal of Obesity* 32, no. 4 (September 2008), 536-41.

14 K.E. Stebbins, C.C. Mose, and M.H. Goldschmidt, "Feline Oral Neoplasia: A Ten-Year Survey," *Veterinary Pathology*, 26, no. 2 (1989): 121–8.

15 Jackie M. Wypij, "A Naturally Occurring Feline Model of Head and Neck Squamous Cell Carcinoma," *Pathology Research International* 2013, no. 502197 (June 2013), http://dx.doi.org/10.1155/2013/502197.

16 Ibid.

17 L.A. Snyder et al., "p53 Expression and Environmental Tobacco
    Smoke Exposure in Feline Oral Squamous Cell Carcinoma,"
    Veterinary Pathology 41, no. 3 (May 2004), 209-14.

18 Elizabeth R. Bertone, Laura A. Snyder, and Antony S. Moore,
    "Environmental Tobacco Smoke and Risk of Malignant Lymphoma
    in Pet Cats," *American Journal of Epidemiology* 156, no. 3 (April 2002),
    268-73.

19 Janeen H. Trembley et al., "Emergence of Protein Kinase CK2 as a
    Key Target in Cancer Therapy," *Biofactors* 36, no. 3 (May-June 2010),
    187-95.

Chapter 9

1   Hywel Williams and Andres Pembroke, "Sniffer Dogs in the
    Melanoma Clinic?" *The Lancet* 333, no. 8640, (April 1989): 734.

2   György Horvath et al., "Human Ovarian Carcinomas Detected by
    Specific Odor," *Integrative Cancer Therapies* 7, no. 2 (June 2008): 76-80.

3   American Cancer Society, "Survival Rates for Ovarian Cancer, by
    Stage," http://www.cancer.org/cancer/ovariancancer/detailedguide/
    ovarian-cancer-survival-rates.

4   "Survival Rates for Stomach Cancer, by Stage,"
    http://www.cancer.org/cancer/stomachcancer/detailedguide/
    stomach-cancer-survival-rates.

5   Tomoyuki Yada Chizu Yokoi, and Naomi Uemura, "The Current
    State of Diagnosis and Treatment for Early Gastric Cancer,"
    Diagnostic and Therapeutic Endoscopy 2013, no. 241320 (2013),
    http://www.hindawi.com/journals/dte/2013/241320/.

6   Giuseppe Lippi and Gianfranco Cervellin, "Canine Olfactory
    Detection of Cancer Versus Laboratory Testing: Myth or Opportunity?"
    Clinical Chemistry and Laboratory Medicine 50, no. 3 (2012): 435-9.

7   Peter Tyson, "Dogs' Dazzling Sense of Smell," *Nova scienceNOW* (2012)
    http://www.pbs.org/wgbh/nova/nature/dogs-sense-of-smell.html.

8   Lippi, Cervellin, "Canine Olfactory Detection of Cancer."

9   Ibid.

10 G. Konvalina and H. Haick, "Sensors for Breath Testing: From
    Nanomaterials to Comprehensive Disease Detection," *Accounts of
    Chemical Research* 47, no. 1 (2013): 66-76.

11   World Health Organization, "Screening for Various Cancers,"
     http://www.who.int/cancer/detection/variouscancer/en/.

12   Gould M.K. et al., "Accuracy of Positron Emission Tomography
     for Diagnosis of Pulmonary Nodules and Mass Lesions: a Meta-
     analysis," *Journal of the American Medical Association*, 285
     (September-October 2001): 914–24.

13   Roberto F. Machado et al., "Detection of Lung Cancer by
     Sensor Array Analyses of Exhaled Breath," *American Journal
     of Respiratory and Critical Care Medicine* 171, no 11 (2005): 1286–91.

14   R. Ehmann et al., "Canine Scent Detection in the Diagnosis of Lung
     Cancer: Revisiting a Puzzling Phenomenon," *European Respiratory
     Journal* 39, no. 3 (March 2012): 669-76.

15   Robert T. Gordon et al., "The Use of Canines in the Detection of
     Human Cancer," *Journal of Alternative and Complementary Medicine*
     14, no. 1 (January-February 2008): 61-7.

16   Z.Q. Xu et al., "A Nanomaterial-Based Breath Test for Distinguishing
     Gastric Cancer from Benign Gastric Conditions," *British Journal of
     Cancer* 108, no. 4 (March 2013): 941-50.

17   Caroline Halwick, "Gastric Cancer Detected in a Breath Test," *The
     ASCO Post* 5, no. 10 (June 25, 2014), http://www.ascopost.com/issues/
     june-25,-2014/gastric-cancer-detected-in-a-breath-test.aspx.

18   Nir Peled et al., "Non-invasive Breath Analysis of Pulmonary
     Nodules," *Journal of Thoracic Oncology* 7, no. 10 (October 2012):
     1528-33.

19   Nir Peled et al., "Volatile Fingerprints of Cancer Specific Genetic
     Mutations," *Nanomedicine: Nanotechnology, Biology, and Medicine* 9,
     no. 6 (August 2013): 758–66.

20   Michael McCulloch et al., "Diagnostic Accuracy of Canine Scent
     Detection in Early- and Late-Stage Lung and Breast Cancers,"
     Integrative Cancer Therapies 5, no. 1 (March 2006): 1-10.

21   National Institutes of Health, "A Timeline of Pregnancy Testing."
     http://history.nih.gov/exhibits/thinblueline/timeline.html#1970.

22   UCLA Department of Epidemiology, "International
     Controversies in HIV/AIDS Control,"
     http://www.ph.ucla.edu/epi/controversies_hiv.html.

23   FDA, "Approval of First In-Home Rapid HIV Antibody Test Kit,"
     July 3, 2012, http://www.fda.gov/ForConsumers/ConsumerUpdates/
     ucm310545.htm.

24   FDA warning letter to 23andMe CEO Ann Wojcicki, November
     22, 2013, http://www.fda.gov/iceci/enforcementactions/
     warningletters/2013/ucm376296.htm.

25   Carolyn M. Willis et al., "Olfactory Detection of Human Bladder
     Cancer by Dogs: Proof of Principle Study," *British Medical Journal* 329,
     no. 712 (September 2004), http://www.bmj.com/content/329/7468/712.

Chapter 10

1   Erez Erlichman, "Labrador Most Popular Dog in Israel,"
     Ynetnews.com, June 23, 2011,
     http://www.ynetnews.com/articles/0,7340,L-4074841,00.html.

2   American Pet Products Association, "Pet Industry Market Size &
     Ownership Statistics," http://www.americanpetproducts.org/press_
     industrytrends.asp.

3   Centers for Disease Control and Prevention, "History of One Health,"
     http://www.cdc.gov/onehealth/people-events.html.

4   Eyal Klement et al., "'One Health,' from science to policy: examples
     from the Israeli experience," *Veterinaria Italiana*, 45, no. 1 (January–
     March 2009): 45–53.

5   Doron Kopelman et al., "Magnetic resonance–guided focused
     ultrasound surgery (MRgFUS). Four ablation treatments of a single
     canine hepatocellular adenoma," *HPB (Oxford)* 8, no. 4 (2006): 292-8.

6   N. Yamamoto et al., "Immunotherapy of Metastatic Breast Cancer
     Patients with Vitamin D-Binding Protein-Derived Macrophage
     Activating Factor (GcMAF)," *International Journal of Cancer* 122,
     no. 2 (January 2008): 461-7; "Immunotherapy of Metastatic
     Colorectal Cancer with Vitamin D-Binding Protein-Derived
     Macrophage-Activating Factor, GcMAF," *Cancer Immunology,
     Immunotherapy* 57, no. 7 (July 2008): 1007-16; "Immunotherapy for
     Prostate Cancer with Gc Protein-Derived Macrophage-Activating
     Factor, GcMAF," *Translational Oncology* 1, no. 2 (July 2008): 65-72.

7   American Cancer Society, "Pancreatic Cancer Survival by Stage,"
    http://www.cancer.org/cancer/pancreaticcancer/detailedguide/
    pancreatic-cancer-survival-rates.

8   American Cancer Society, "What are the survival rates for
    colorectal cancer by stage?" http://www.cancer.org/cancer/
    colonandrectumcancer/detailedguide/colorectal-cancer-survival-rates.

9   American Cancer Society, "Survival Rates for Stomach Cancer by
    Stage," http://www.cancer.org/cancer/stomachcancer/detailedguide/
    stomach-cancer-survival-rates.

Chapter 11

1   World Cancer Research Fund International, "Stomach Cancer
    Statistics," http://www.wcrf.org/cancer_statistics/data_specific_
    cancers/stomach_cancer_statistics.php.

2   Anne Sauer et al., "School of Medicine, 1893," *Concise Encyclopedia of
    Tufts History.*

3   Stanford Health Care, "Hereditary Diffuse Gastric Cancer
    Syndrome (CDH1),"
    https://stanfordhealthcare.org/medical-conditions/cancer/hdgc.html.

4   A.K. Patnaik, A.I. Hurvitz, and G.F. Johnson, "Canine Gastric
    Adenocarcinoma," *Veterinary Pathology* 15 (1978): 600-607.

5   National Canine Cancer Foundation, "Gastric Cancer,"
    http://www.wearethecure.org/gastric-cancer.

6   Tonje Seim-Wikse et al., "Breed Predisposition to Canine Gastric
    Carcinoma — a Study Based on the Norwegian Canine Cancer
    Register," *Acta Veterinaria Scandinavica* 55, no. 25 (March 2013),
    http://www.actavetscand.com/content/55/1/25.

7   World Health Organization International Agency for Research on
    Cancer, Helicobacter pylori Eradication as a Strategy for Preventing
    Gastric Cancer. http://www.iarc.fr/en/publications/pdfs-online/wrk/
    wrk8/Helicobacter_pylori_Eradication.pdf.

8   National Cancer Institute, "Helicobacter pylori and Cancer,"
    http://www.cancer.gov/cancertopics/factsheet/Risk/h-pylori-cancer.

9   Linda Morris Brown, "Helicobacter pylori: Epidemiology and Routes
    of Transmission," *Epidemiologic Reviews* 22, no. 2 (2000): 283-97.

10 Tufts University Cummings School of Veterinary Medicine, "Foster Hospital for Small Animals at Tufts," http://vet.tufts.edu/foster-hospital-small-animals/about-us/.

11 Tufts University Cummings School of Veterinary Medicine, "About the Tufts Wildlife Clinic," http://vet.tufts.edu/tufts-wildlife-clinic/about-the-clinic/.

12 National Cancer Institute, "Brief History of Cancer Registration," http://training.seer.cancer.gov/registration/registry/history/.

13 Statistics Canada, "About the Canadian Cancer Registry, http://www.statcan.gc.ca/pub/82-231-x/2010001/part-partie1-eng.htm.

Epilogue

1   The Ohio State University Veterinary Medical Center, "New cancer drug for dogs benefits human research," September 23, 2014, http://vet.osu.edu/vmc-news/new-cancer-drug-dogs-benefits-human-research.

2   Andy Hyland, "Dogs may be the key to discovering new treatments for osteosarcoma," *KU Medical Center News*, April 28, 2014, http://www.kumc.edu/news-listing-page/testing-new-drugs-for-osteosarcoma.html.

3   MD Anderson Cancer Center, "MD Anderson Announces Collaboration with Johnson & Johnson Innovation on cancer immunotherapy," January 21, 2014, http://www.mdanderson.org/newsroom/news-releases/2014/cancer-immunotherapy.html.

4   Novartis, "Novartis announces CTL019 data published in *NEJM* demonstrating efficacy in certain patients with acute lymphoblastic leukemia (ALL)," October 15, 2014, https://www.novartis.com/news/media-releases/novartis-announces-ctl019-data-published-nejm-demonstrating-efficacy-certain.